Compresses and
Other Therapeutic Applications

Compresses

and Other

Therapeutic Applications

A Handbook from
the Ita Wegman Clinic

Monika Fingado

Floris Books

Translated by Tessa Therkleson (PhD, RN)
and Sarah Therkleson (BN, RN)
Illustrations by Gabriela de Carvalho

First published in 2001 by as *Therapeutische Wickel und
Kompressen – Handbuch aus der Ita Wegman Klinik*
This English edition published in 2012 by Floris Books

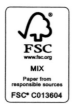

FSC
www.fsc.org
MIX
Paper from
responsible sources
FSC® C013604

British Library CIP Data available

ISBN 978-086315-875-9

Printed in Great Britain
by CPI Group (UK) Ltd, Croydon

Contents

Foreword

For thousands of years, compresses, washes, oils and
ointments have belonged to the healing treasures of
all cultures. These external applications are applied
directly on the skin to ease illnesses and treat wounds.
In ancient healing, warming and cooling of the body
using applications had a significant role. As medicine
has become focused on the scientific evidence of the
substance, external applications to the skin have become
less popular, possibly because it is not so easy to calculate
the quantity of substance being absorbed.

In European folk medicine, we still find therapeutic
applications such as compresses. Many adults experienced in childhood chest and back compresses that
bring back memories of aroma, warmth and nurture.
Anthroposophical medicine as developed by Rudolf
Steiner and Ita Wegman considers external applications have an important place in both the hospital and
home. External applications are used for skin conditions,
wounds and infectious illness, even to support critically
ill people on life support. Monika Fingado has compiled
the most significant and relevant external applications
collected throughout ninety years of experience in
the first anthroposophical hospital in Europe, the Ita
Wegman Clinic in Arlesheim, Switzerland. Tessa and
Sarah Therkleson must be thanked for translating this
book and enabling English-speaking readers to access
this valued resource.

Therapeutic external applications are part of a world-
wide renaissance and rediscovery of ancient healing
methods. Since its founding, anthroposophical medicine
has integrated external applications naturally into its
healing approach because this medicine comes from
a holistic understanding of diagnosis and treatment.

In this respect, it is significant whether a substance is absorbed through the digestion, blood, lungs or skin. An application that is absorbed through the skin is always connected with intense awareness and sensory perception, whereas oral medicines are perceived only by the senses of taste and touch in the mouth, the remaining process then becoming unconscious. This difference becomes very obvious, when striving to apply scientific cause and effect to the understanding of external applications. A blind study is hardly possible if the recipient is acutely conscious of the experience. External treatments activate specific sensations through the stimulation of warmth, cold and touch. It is these aspects of the external application that are especially important in establishing indications.

In general, three aspects differentiate external applications: substance, the medium and the caring approach of the provider. The substance may be a plant extract such as ginger, a mineral substance such as copper or an animal substance such as honey. The medium may be a warm, cold, dry or moist application. The caring approach is conveyed through an attitude of attentiveness, nurture and calm. These three processes continually interrelate and can be modified in a number of ways; for example by changing the duration, frequency, rhythm, time of day and by combining with another medicinal substance or treatment. External applications may also be modified by being given in combination with another medicinal treatment. It is important that changes to treatments are indicated as different external applications emphasise different processes; for example, the substance is the most important part of the treatment in a mustard compress. Mustard releases a powerful warmth activity onto the skin. In contrast the most significant process of the yarrow compress is the moist warm medium used. For the rhythmic einreibung* the

---

* Rhythmic einreibung is a form of massage used in anthroposophical nursing. Its techniques were developed by the physician Margarethe Hauschka, based on suggestions by Ita Wegman. See Fingado's companion book, *Rhythmic Einreibung.*

most important process is the intention of encompassing and caring for the recipient.

The effect of external applications can be understood from three different perspectives: physical, soul and life energy. Through different sensory experiences the recipient's awareness is directed to their body, bringing a positive experience and valuing of their whole body. On the soul level the recipient experiences relaxation and release of tension that enables an emotional and physical breathing out. Memories may be awoken; sometimes traumatic experiences can be activated. The recipient may even enter a relaxed, dreamy, fanciful state. Life energy and self healing may be stimulated through the use of warm or cold substances; processes of circulation, breathing, excretion, regeneration are enhanced, and pain often alleviated.

This book places a special emphasis on how medicinal substances are presented. A close relationship with the medicinal substance is essential in providing the indications. Specific substances derived from plants, animals and minerals are interrelated and connected to other substances, to processes of metamorphosis, to the seasons and cosmic rhythms. The loving, sensitive phenomenological observation and descriptions of the plants are more relevant in this situation than a functional, analytical method. This way of looking at the world reflects the fundamental gesture of nursing that is less focused on acute intervention and rather on development and growth processes of the patient.

In this sense we wish this book to be shared with nurses and physicians interested in external applications, in order to develop their practice by using these healing methods.

Rolf Heine
Co-ordinator of the
International Forum for Anthroposophic Nurses
Filderstadt, Germany

Translators' note

The English version of this book developed in a manner similar to the companion book, *Rhythmic Einreibung*. A dialogue evolved between two anthroposophic nurses: Tessa who was educated in New Zealand, and Sarah who was educated at the Filderklinik in Germany. The translation developed over four years and included regular dialogue and consultation with the author. Additional indications for treatments and further references have been included where appropriate. We would like to especially acknowledge the support given by Weleda New Zealand Ltd and the constant encouragement and guidance of Godfrey Therkleson.

Preface

*A plant is like a self-willed human being, out of which
we can obtain all we desire, if we only treat it in its
own way.*

Goethe, *Elective Affinities*

External applications from plant substance can have
a number of different outcomes and effects such as
pain relief, relaxation, stimulation, revitalization and
self healing. In order for the healing process to work,
each medicinal plant needs to be considered holisti-
cally, ideally using an approach that encompasses exact
observation and in-depth understanding. A Goethean
approach applies a fresh perspective towards observing
the nature of each plant that enables its inner qualities to
be revealed. For example, oxalis grows in shaded forest
areas and is used very differently to the sunlight-loving
camomile. Oxalis would not be used as a hot compress,
such as camomile as the heat would restrict the release
of its inherent qualities.

The anthroposophical understanding of the human
being and nature provides ways to appreciating the
healing qualities and effects of plants as well as those
obtained from mineral and animal substances. When
external applications are used with this awareness, they
provide a real service towards a healing response in the
patient. Such a therapeutic approach reflects the Greek
word *therapeia* meaning service and care.

This book strives to support this process. It evolved
out of an internal manual developed at the Ita Wegman
Clinic in Arlesheim, Switzerland, following years of
experience of the medical team.

External applications have an important part to play
in nursing practice. Through the nurses' experience

and observation of the patient, they are encouraged to develop their confidence and competence in their area of expertise. Collaboration between the nurse and physician enables external applications to be selected with the greatest therapeutic effect.

Special acknowledgement is extended to the following nurses at the Ita Wegman Clinic, who supported the preparation of this book: Anette Beisswenger, Elisabeth Gold, Brigitte Greve, Gisela Hager, Christiane Radlingmayr, Mechthild Renz, Marianne Scheurer and Silvia Stockler.

The active use of external applications may create fresh discoveries and questions that lead to new treatments. This makes this book an unfinished work. All users of this handbook are encouraged to continue their own voyage of discovery and research.

Monika Fingado

1

Background

Important guidelines

The difference between wrapping-cloths, cloths and compresses is that a wrapping-cloth encompasses the entire torso, while a cloth and compress is on a specific part such as an organ. Almost all cloths and compresses also require a wrapping-cloth around the body as part of the treatment.

Options and boundaries
Many of the external applications are able to be done in the home, where they can be of enormous help. Some may even be self applied. Readers are encouraged to consider the indications and contra-indications provided. These treatments are not a substitute for medical advice. A physician is necessary if there is any uncertainty around the cause of the condition, or the symptoms do not disappear following the appropriate application. External applications can be a complementary therapy alongside other more conventional treatments. Even in acute life-threatening illnesses they may have a significant, supportive and therapeutic role.

Questions for the recipient
Each external application can be a question to the recipient, and the response of the body or soul is an expression of the individual's answer. If the nurse or practitioner carries a strong image of the substance and its power then this question is carried with increased clarity, and the effect on the recipient is more apparent. Such an approach enables the giver to have a clearer sense of understanding and direction

To some extent, a compress can be adapted according to the individual need and experience of time, temperature and potency. It is important that the basic fundamental process of the application is not compromised or prevented from being effective. For example, if a person is given a camomile abdominal compress that is ideally applied as hot as possible, but they cannot tolerate it at more than body temperature, then the treatment cannot be fully effective. If in the subsequent session the temperature still cannot be increased, then there is a question about the appropriateness of the application. Perhaps a new substance or a different external application is required.

Answers from the recipient

A full response from the recipient should not be expected too early. A yarrow liver compress may result in a number of different effects many hours later, such as increased alertness, deep tiredness, desperate hunger, thirst or increased urinary output.

Sometimes the recipient becomes more conscious through the intense warmth of the application such that the response comes from deep within and results in a previously unknown need or feeling. It is especially important to be awake and aware of these responses as they express what is happening for the recipient in a given situation. Some people are very aware of their different experiences, which they differentiate quite specifically, while others will require the nurse to be more observant.

The recipient and the surroundings

In order that the recipient is prepared for the question, they need to be informed of the goal and process of the external application, as is appropriate with all treatments. They must also be prepared to be open to the treatment so that it is able to work for them.

Prior to each treatment, the recipient needs to be in comfortable clothing and should go to the toilet. Air the room and clear it of any disturbances such as telephone, radio or direct sunlight. Ideally, place a note outside the room indicating not to disturb while the treatment is in progress.

Preparation of the external application is done either in the room or nearby, depending on available space and the recipient's situation. It is often appropriate for a tea to be prepared near the recipient or a lemon to be cut such that the etheric oils can be inhaled. Nonetheless, the area around the recipient needs to be free of clutter. In the discussion on the cloths and compresses, the compresses are usually soaked directly next to the recipient, while the wrapping-cloths and hot-waterbottles are prepared in another space.

After the compress is applied, the cloths are straightened over the body part being treated so the recipient can rest comfortably, with the outer blanket drawn up to encompass the shoulders. It is important that the recipient has warm feet during the treatment, as this aids relaxation. A hot-waterbottle at the feet is generally not ideal as awareness is drawn to two different parts of the body — to the feet and to the part being treated. It is preferable that the recipient has a hot-waterbottle or footbath prior to the treatment or wears warm socks during the treatment. In order that the recipient is relaxed while lying on their back, a knee roll may be required or the recipient may be more comfortable resting on their side.

Time and rhythm
The application has to be included in the daily routine, and sufficient time following the treatment must be allowed for rest and stillness. After an external application, it is important to have a rest time that enables the person to respond appropriately. In the rest time, disturbances need to be minimised. Apart from some exceptions such as the mustard footbath for a headache, a series of applications are generally given before a full response can be expected. Repeated treatments stimulate awareness and differentiation of the body enabling a more conscious answer to the question.

Rhythm carries life is a response that Rudolf Steiner gave towards understanding the essence of life. Ideally, a treatment is given regularly at the same time of the day so that a sense of healthy rhythm is carried by the recipient. As with any rhythmical activity a pause is important; this is the reason we have a rest day between courses of treatments, when giving external applications. On the day following the rest day, a sense of rebirth may be experienced and the treatment does not simply become a habit. After four or at most eight weeks the external application should be stopped. Depending on the situation, the treatment series may be repeated again after a break. The anabolic and self-healing processes run in a four-weekly rhythm. If this is taken into account the self-healing processes are more effectively supported.

Warmth

Warmth carries an essential role in all external applications. Warmth that can permeate and bring everything into movement is required for all development and healing. For example, it is only when we 'warm to an idea' that we can respond and become an active participant.

Depending on the substance, a variety of completely different warmth qualities are applied. An oil compress activates a soft, encompassing warmth, a mustard compress creates an aggressive warmth effect, while a warm moist compress stimulates an inner intense warmth. In all applications, whenever a specific part of the body is warmed or cooled, the whole organism is being addressed and involved.

When applying an external application, it is necessary to ensure the recipient does not lie uncovered for too long and during the treatment warmth is maintained evenly. After the treatment, the recipient needs to gradually acclimatise to the changed temperature outside the treatment room.

Required materials

Cloths for external applications are made from natural absorbent fabric that is breathable and malleable with a soft feel, and not from artificial fibres. These factors are essential for the effectiveness of the compress. In the Ita Wegman Clinic a variety of specially made compress cloths are prepared. Towels, face-cloths, brushed cotton and flannelette sheeting may be improvised. For example, bed linen may be recycled to make compresses, while the woollen outer cloth may be prepared from a woollen scarf, sock, blanket or jumper (sweater).

Inner cloth
The inner cloth is made from cotton, linen or heavy cotton silk. For moist cloths and compresses the inner cloth is folded into a number of layers until it is the required size. This added bulk allows it to better hold moisture and temperature.

Usually the inner cotton cloth is 40 × 120 cm (16 × 48 in). For many compresses, such as for the stomach, liver and kidney areas the cloth is folded to 20 × 30 cm (8 × 12 in), so there may be eight layers of fabric. When the full sized cotton cloth is folded in half lengthwise it is a suitable size for a body, chest or calf compress. For a smaller compress, such as heart or pulse compress a small face-cloth or cotton cloth may be used.

For a small or large mustard compress use a special mustard cloth. This compress cloth (30 × 120 cm, 12 × 48 in) is a bag folded from the top to the bottom and sewn up the sides to retain the powder. There is an opening at the top to add the mustard powder, rather like a long and narrow pillow case. If desired, a large folded cotton cloth could also be used.

Breast compresses are oval shaped, with a number of layers. They need to be large enough to cover the whole breast area and have an opening around the nipple.

Oil, cream, paste and ointment cloths are made from cotton material, such as used bed linen that has been prepared to the required size.

Wringing-cloth

For hot, wet applications, a wringing-cloth is used to squeeze out the inner cloth. This needs to be about 10 to 15 cm (4–6 in) larger than the inner cloth. Typically, a tea towel is used because it is absorbent and made out of strong cotton cloth.

Outer cloth

Generally, the treated part of the body is wrapped in an outer cloth. The outer cloth needs to be large enough to generously cover the appropriate body part and extend over the inner cloth about 4–5 cm (2 in). The outer cloth is prepared out of comfortable, warm material.

Wool is used for moist applications such as those prepared from tea or lotions, when the warmth needs to be retained as long as possible. Wool has a strong warmth effect and retains the fluid without cooling through evaporation. Soft flannel, molleton cloth or brushed towelling may also be used if wool is unavailable.

Brushed cotton or towelling cloth is used for quark and mustard applications because wool would absorb the substance becoming hardened, discoloured and smelly.

Cream and oil compresses and others such as kaolin, bolus alba and lemon require cotton or flannel wool.

Intermediate cloth

As an outer woollen cloth can be itchy and irritable it is generally covered by an intermediate cloth prepared from soft cotton. The intermediate cloth rests on the skin rather than the woollen cloth.

Resting cloth

A resting cloth is used after some compresses. This is prepared from a soft material that retains the warmth such as heavy cotton flannel or molleton cloth.

Fastener

The method of fastening depends on the type of compress, the substance being used, and the area being treated. Usually a cotton cloth is used to secure the inner cloth, but a scarf, bandage, hat singlet or sock may be more suitable.

Hot-waterbottle
A hot–waterbottle is required for most external applications. It is important that the hot–waterbottle covers the inner cloth for moist, hot and warm applications. The hot–waterbottle rests against the outer cloth such that it lies close to the treated area, without touching it for a satisfactory warming effect. The bottle should be made out of a soft flat rubber; that is only half filled with hot (not boiling) water, and lies flat with no air pockets in it. For hygienic reasons use a soft, comfortable cover that can be changed between patients.

In European hospitals, Fashy hot–waterbottles are used because they are made from high quality, long lasting material.

Bed protection
Bed protection is required for a few compresses, such as fever compresses and those made from mustard, quark or Bolus alba. Ideally, a bed protection is made of thick towelling or plastic sheeting.

Additional utensils
A bowl, spatula, knife, grater, wooden board may need to be used in some applications. These are described, when appropriate under the relevant application. Following use these need to be well cleaned in either a dish washer or with an effective liquid detergent.

Size and quantities
Generally, the amounts given are for an average sized adult. For tea and lotion applications about 300 ml (10 fl oz) needs to be absorbed by the inner cloth, with little or none left over. A measuring spoon, medicine cup, syringe or a bottle lid is used to measure lotions and teas. A teaspoon is 5 ml, the lids on the 100 ml and 200 ml bottles hold 6 ml, while a 50 ml bottle lid holds 4 ml.

Moist hot and warm cloths and compresses

Moist hot compresses are the most frequently used external applications. In these applications, the inner cloth is soaked in a fluid as hot as possible and wrung out before being placed on the body. Generally, moist warm applications don't require a wringing–cloth, and have the same procedure as hot external applications. There are a number of factors to take note of in the preparation and application of cloths and compresses. The following sections offer more in–depth descriptions and details.

Effect

The hot moist compress is intensely warming. It increases circulation, dilates blood vessels and relaxes and releases muscular tension and cramp. Even a compress prepared in warm water has a positive therapeutic effect. The general warming effect is specific and therapeutically focused depending on the selection of lotion, plant or other substance

Liver, abdominal and kidney compresses

Cloth preparation

The inner cloth is folded to the correct size, rolled up and placed inside the wringing–cloth. The wringing–cloth needs to extend 10–15 cm (4–6 in) either side of the inner cloth.

Roll the inner cloth in the wringing–cloth.

The outer cloths consist of two separate cloths, a soft cotton cloth inside a woollen cloth. Lay the soft cot-

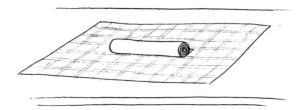

ton cloth on top of the woollen cloth and roll both together
from the outer edge into the
middle. Lay a hot-waterbottle in
the centre to warm both these
cloths.

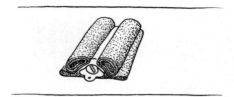

Soaking the inner cloth
Place the wringing–cloth with the inner cloth inside
in a bowl, and pour the hot tea, lotion or mixture over
it. The hot fluid can be poured into the bowl first if
desired.

Keep the ends of the wringing–cloth dry so that they
are easily wrung.

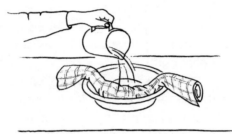

Wringing inner cloth
The moist inner cloth needs to be wrung out very well,
so it can be applied as hot as possible because dry heat
is more tolerable than wet heat. A well wrung cloth
results in minimal cooling and evaporation avoiding the
negative experience of cold and damp. Practitioners,
with heat sensitive hands can
use rubber gloves to wring out
the cloths.

If preparation is in another
room, put the wringing-cloth
with the inner cloth on the hot-
waterbottle warming the outer
cloths and immediately take it
all as a package to the recipient.

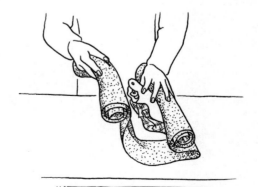

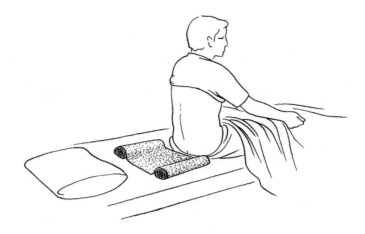

Application of abdominal and liver compress

The recipient sits up and the upper body clothing is lifted to expose the area being treated. It is important that the clothing does not become wet or caught in the outer cloths.

The outer cloths are rolled out behind the back and the recipient lies back on them.

To maintain the warmth of the inner cloth quickly remove it from the wringing–cloth and hold it over the area to be treated, applying it to the skin with dabbing motions to allow gradual tolerance. Once the recipient indicates acceptance of the compress temperature, place it on the skin. Immediately wrap the outer cloth around the torso to prevent further cooling.

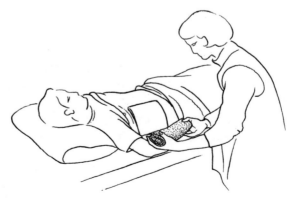

Liver compress

Wrap the outer cloths flat and firmly avoiding folds at the edges, where air can be trapped. Rearranged clothing comfortably and place a light hot–waterbottle over the compress area to maintain warmth. Place a pillow or roll under the knees to relax the stomach muscles; this is especially important if there is pain or discomfort of the stomach.

Application of kidney compress
The recipient sits up and the clothing is lifted to expose the area being treated. It is important that the clothing does not become wet or caught in the outer cloths.

Roll out the outer cloths behind the back. Immediately after removing from the wringing–cloth, lay the inner cloth on the outer cloths.

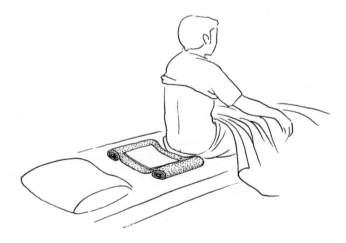

Gently dab the hot inner cloth together with the outer cloth over the kidney region to allow gradual tolerance on the skin. Once the recipient indicates acceptance, place the compress on the skin (see overleaf).

Then the recipient lies down and the outer cloth is immediately drawn around the torso so there is no further cooling.

Wrap the outer cloths flat and firmly avoiding folds at the edges, where air can be trapped. If hot–waterbottles are required, they must have only a small quantity of

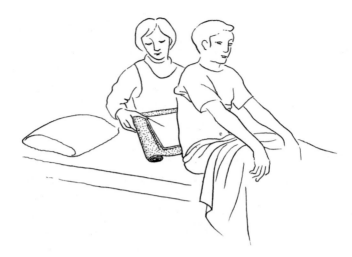

hot water. Lay one on each side of the spine. A pillow must be placed under the small of the back if it is hollow, ensuring the compress is held against the skin and maintains its warmth.

Finishing off
Remove the damp inner and outer cloths, cover the recipient leave them to rest with a hot-waterbottle if needed. This allows the intense warmth activated in the treatment to gradually dissipate.

Wash the inner cloth with warm water, rinse and hang to dry with the other cloths. The cloths can be used a number of times, rewashing as needed.

Body and chest compress

The body and chest compress is best applied with two people assisting because the cloth is thin and can cool down quickly. When the compress is applied evenly it is experienced as comfortable and pleasant. If this is not done the compress cools down too quickly and is experienced as unpleasant and the treatment is counter-productive. Good preparation and rapid application are especially important for this compress.

Cloth preparation

Fold the inner cloth to the correct size, roll up and place inside the wringing-cloth. The wringing-cloth needs to extend 10–15 cm (4–6 in) on either side of the inner cloth.

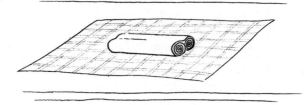

Roll the inner cloth in the wringing-cloth.

The outer cloths consist of two separate cloths, a soft cotton cloth inside a woollen cloth. Lay the soft cotton cloth on top of the woollen cloth and roll both together from the outer edge into the middle. Lay a hot-waterbottle in the centre to warm both these cloths.

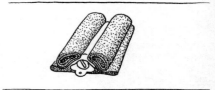

Soaking the inner cloth

Place the wringing-cloth with the inner cloth inside in a bowl, and pour the hot tea, lotion or mixture over it. The hot fluid can be poured into the bowl first if desired.

Keep the ends of the wringing-cloth dry so that they are easily wrung.

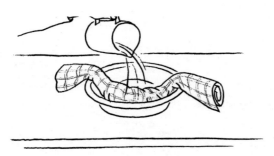

Wringing inner cloth

The moist inner cloth needs to be wrung out very well, so it can be applied as hot as possible because dry heat is more tolerable than wet heat. A well wrung cloth results in minimal cooling and evaporation avoiding the negative experience of cold and damp. Practitioners, with heat sensitive hands can use rubber gloves to wring out the cloths.

If preparation is in another room, put the wringing-cloth with the inner cloth on the hot-waterbottle warming the outer cloths and immediately take it all as a package to the recipient.

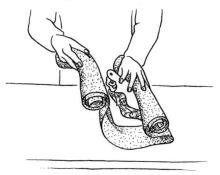

Application of the body and chest compress

The recipient sits up and the clothing is lifted to expose the area being treated. It is important that the clothing does not become wet or caught in the outer cloths.

Roll out the outer cloths behind the back. Immediately after removing from the wringing-cloth, lay the inner cloth on the outer cloths.

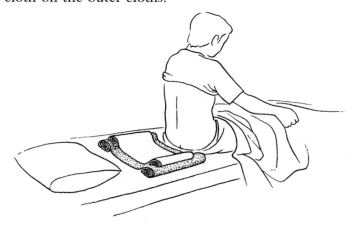

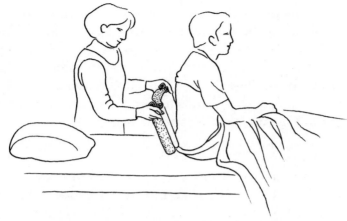

Gently dab the hot inner cloth together with the outer cloth to allow gradual tolerance and preparation of the recipient. Once the recipient indicates acceptance, place the compress on the skin, and let the recipient lie down.

Application with two people: one person stands to the left and the other to the right of the recipient. Unroll the inner cloth to each side and apply as hot as is tolerated. Then quickly wrap the outer cloth around and tuck in firmly, avoiding folds at the edges, where air can be trapped.

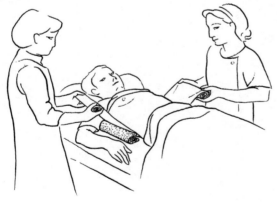

Application with one person: unroll the inner cloth on one side applying as hot as is tolerated. Quickly cover with the outer cloth. Then complete the other side in the same way and draw the outer cloth firmly around the body.

Rearrange clothing so it is comfortable and without lumps under the recipient. Place a pillow or roll under the knees to relax the stomach muscles, this is especially important, when there is pain or discomfort in the abdomen. A pillow can be placed under the small of the back if it is hollow. This ensures the compress is held against the skin and maintains its warmth.

Finishing off
Remove the damp inner and outer cloths, cover the recipient and leave them to rest with a hot-waterbottle if needed. This allows the intense warmth activated in the treatment to gradually dissipate.

Wash the inner cloth with warm water, rinse and hang to dry with the other cloths. The cloths can be used a number of times, rewashing as needed.

The effect of medicinal plants

Most compresses are prepared with plant substances, so a short explanation of the significance of plant observation is given to assist in understanding this therapeutic effect. Fundamental terms that have evolved out of the anthroposophical understanding of the human being and anthroposophical medicine are used to enable a more comprehensive appreciation of this therapeutic approach. Suggestions for further reading are at the end of the book.

The threefold plant

The plant grows between the earth and cosmos and comprises root, flower and leaf. The roots extend deep in the tough, hard earth. The fine fibrous roots absorb the minerals. Through this activity the roots are completely bound to physical, earthly laws. The roots are the plant's densest substance. In the mineral world this is characterised by salt. Rudolf Steiner described the roots as being totally beholden to the earth, even becoming slaves to the earth.[1]

The developing shoot that grows towards the sun, evolves from the earthly watery realm into the airy warm environment above. Through growth the plant is drawn out and upwards toward the air and warmth, with substance entering solution and form becoming lighter, more refined and differentiated. As the plant develops the leaves normally become smaller and more contracted, while the flower expands releasing its pollen and aroma to the environment. The plant opens totally to the light and warmth above, absorbing and transforming these elements into the volatile etheric oils.

In the mineral world sulfur represents the substance that contains the most intense warmth and heat, such that it burns. Sulfur heat and energy are pure forms of warmth. The warmth energy of the flower, as contained in the etheric oils, is described as a sulfuric process. The opposite process occurs in the roots, which is seen through the clear, translucent salt crystals transformed from the earth.

You could say that the plant is most plant-like in the green leaf and stem. In the leaf and stem the plant breaths, and obtains energy in the processes of photosynthesis. This middle area of the plant is arranged rhythmically between stem and leaf, with the stem being long and thin and the leaf flat and broad. The stem is differentiated through having a series of nodes. There is a condensing and releasing of energy in a continual repetitive exchange.

This part of the plant can be described as the mercurial part. The liquid metal mercury has the quality of being able to divide into numerous drops that quickly draw back into one large drop.

As each plant grows it works with the qualities inherent in root, flower and leaf developing its own inner form and characteristics. Sometimes a plant manifests extreme development in one aspect; this one-sidedness can be seen as a possibility for a therapeutic effect. One-sided qualities in a plant are sometimes expressed in an unexpected manner, for example the hot sulfuric forces that are normally in the flower in the Cruciferae family can be found both in the seed of the mustard and the root of the horseradish.

A plant that dominates in the middle region may have a balancing, harmonising effect between the polar opposite energies of the flower and the root.

The functional threefoldness of the human being
These plant qualities of sulfur, salt and mercury are also working within the human being.

The metabolic system reflects the sulfur forces of warming, moving, releasing energies, which are especially found in the digestive organs and the muscular system. Rudolf Steiner calls this the metabolic–limb system.

In the brain, nerves and sense organs the metabolic processes are reduced to a minimum. In this part of the body salt forces predominate, with peace, quiet and stillness ruling in order that humans can think. This area is called the nerve–sense system.

The rhythmic system is the rhythmical exchange of

expansion and contraction that is most manifest in the heartbeat and breathing. This is especially observed in the middle part of the body and is known as the rhythmic system. Here is indicated the mercurial quality of holding and letting go, condensing and expanding.

When these three qualities in the different body systems work harmoniously then the human body is healthy. When the releasing/dissolving qualities of the metabolic system are too strong fever may develop, while if the cold hard processes of the head predominate sclerosis or deposits may occur in the body.

The human being in relation to the plant

The functional threefoldness of the human being is related to and compared to that of an upside down plant. If the relationship of the qualities of the human nerve-sense, rhythmic and metabolic-limb systems is considered alongside those of an upside down plant, the similarities indicate that different parts of certain plants can be used therapeutically for human beings. For example, a plant with a strong flowering quality may support the human metabolic system and be used if the hardening nerve-sense forces are overly strong. In such a case, the intense flower qualities have a warming and dissolving effect.

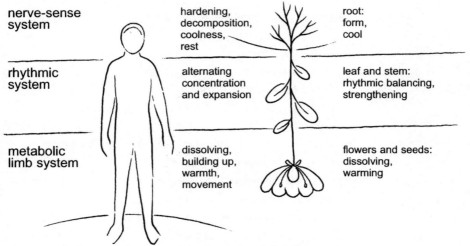

nerve-sense system — hardening, decomposition, coolness, rest — root: form, cool

rhythmic system — alternating concentration and expansion — leaf and stem: rhythmic balancing, strengthening

metabolic limb system — dissolving, building up, warmth, movement — flowers and seeds: dissolving, warming

Comparison between the parts of the human and the plant

The different parts of plant, animal and human
Rudolf Steiner gave a fresh way of understanding the
physical body by considering its different aspects.

The plant develops from the substances it absorbs
from the earth and air enabling it to develop a physical
body. The physical body is permeated with water that
allows it to develop and reproduce a life or etheric body.
If the etheric energy were the only energy in the plant it
would grow continuously leaf by leaf, reproducing itself
endlessly. Through meeting the earth environment the
plant meets very different energies.

The plant grows towards its soul-like part,
which can also be termed the astral body.
The astral body enables it to remain a plant
rather than to be overcome by uncontrolled
movements or feelings. This is because the
plant meets its astral body from above, outside
of itself. The plant's astral body is not bound
to the plant's organs, rather it is externally
connected and acts from the outside.[2]

The flower impulse comes to the fresh green bud
from above. The impulse sinks into the flower arrest-
ing vegetative growth and forming from the outside
the coloured bloom. Because of this, the flower has a
soul-like impression that causes humans to respond with
their soul life. This connection between the flower and
animal is described by Rudolf Steiner in the following
verse:

Look the plant —
It is the earthbound butterfly.
Look the butterfly —
It is the plant released by the cosmos.[3]

A flower sits upon the green bud like a parasite that
lives its life at the expense of another. Without chlo-
rophyll the flower cannot build starch, rather it has
the quality of using energy like the animal. It creates
warmth through the fiery flowering process.

In the vegetative green bud and the coloured flower
polar qualities manifest. In each plant these qualities exist
in a characteristic manner. For example, in camomile

the flowering process is so intense that the vegetative growth becomes quickly arrested. On the other hand, the dandelion has strong vegetative energy that seems to be unaffected by the flower as it keeps developing just as strongly. Rudolf Steiner said poisonous plants have become too connected to animal qualities and they develop empty spaces that store poisonous substances that are end products of their metabolic processes.[4]

Animals and humans have physical and etheric bodies, like the plant. They also have an inner connection to their soul qualities, with their own soul and astral body that enables them to experience emotions, consciousness and the ability to develop an inner space for themselves. The human being possesses above this a fourth body that is their own individual personality. This fourth body gives them their consciousness of self and sense of 'I', and is connected to the blood and warmth organism.

The plant connects the vegetative etheric and blood like astral energy, while the human connects the physical-etheric bodies and the soul-sense of "I" bodies. The interplay between these bodies and how they connect in the human indicates how well incarnated* a person is and how healthy they are.

---

* The Latin word *carne* means flesh.

2

Footbaths

Footbaths are included because they are very effective, convenient and require minimal preparation. Instead of using a bathmilk, a litre (quart) of herbal tea may be used such as lavender flowers or rosemary leaves. Tea preparations for external applications are described further in the text (see page 149). In a deep basin put warm water, with the appropriate bathmilk, tea or lotion. Generally, both the feet and calves are immersed completely in the water.

An alternative to a commercial bathmilk is 4 to 5 drops of an essential oil mixed with a tablespoon of a fatty emulsion, such as milk and added to the footbath.

Copper sulfate (cuprum sulfuricum)

This footbath is included because it is a simple, useful adjunct to managing conditions such as hypertension and/or those with damaged kidneys (Translators).

Indications

Constitutional kidney problems
High blood pressure caused by kidneys
Damaged kidneys from diabetes mellitus

Material

Basin, big enough to cover ankles with water
6 ml copper sulfate 20% lotion
200 ml (7 fl oz) water
Large and small towels
Plastic or rubber gloves

Procedure

Fill the basin with warm water at body temperature; it should be comfortable and not too hot for the recipient. Add the copper sulfate lotion and mix well (wearing gloves).

The recipient sits in a relaxed position for the foot-bath, with the upper legs and hips covered with a large towel to maintain warmth.

Duration 10 minutes, or as long as the footbath is experienced as comfortable.

Finishing off Dry the feet well with the small towel and put on warm socks. Empty the footbath, wash and dry it.

Rest Quarter of an hour

Lavender (Lavendula augustifolia)

Lavender belongs to the warmth loving, aromatic, *Labiatae* family. Its rich etheric oil is especially found in the sweet smelling flowers that grow out of the stalks and reach high above the silvery green leaves.

Lavender has a deep warming, relaxing, calming and harmonizing effect.

The lavender footbath is given at body temperature or a little cooler. The recipient needs to experience the footbath as pleasantly comfortable, with additional warm water added as needed.

Indications Difficulty going to sleep due to nervous restlessness, tension and cramping
Nervous tension, with heart palpitations
Restlessness, with troublesome thoughts

Contra-indications Allergy or over-sensitivity to lavender
Venous complications, such as varicose veins or vein infections like thrombophlebitis
Skin damage or weeping, infected wounds on the legs

Material Basin, large enough to cover calves with water
Bathmilk, 10–15 ml (2–3 tsp)
Large towel

Place water in the basin and add the bathmilk. Mix in **Procedure**
the bathmilk with your hand using a rhythmic lem-
niscate (figure-of-8) movement for about a minute to
re-enliven the water.

The recipient sits in a relaxed position for the footbath, with the upper legs and hips covered by a large
towel to maintain warmth.

The feet are placed in the footbath for 15 to 30
minutes, as long as the footbath is experienced as
comfortable.

Quarter of an hour   **Rest**

Dry the feet well with the small towel and put on warm **Finishing off**
socks. Empty the footbath, wash and dry it.

Lemon (Citrus limonum)

Lemon belongs to the *Rutaceae* family. Probably native
to Central Asia, it has naturalised throughout many parts
of the world always preferring sheltered locations, with
adequate light and warmth. The lemon fruit has a structured ordered form and lemon's etheric oils have warming qualities that are released, when the lemon skin is
pierced. The lemon fruit has a drawing-in tendency that
is refreshing and calming.

The lemon footbath is given at body temperature or
a little cooler.* The recipient needs to experience the
footbath as pleasantly comfortable.

Lack of body warmth often accompanied by cold feet **Indications**
Loss of ability to concentrate such as may occur from
      lack of sleep, disturbed day and night rhythm or
      extreme mental exertion
Agitated breathing caused by hyperventilation, anxiety
      or stress
Lack of a sense of the self

* The lemon footbath is commonly used in Australasia and has been
  added to this translation.

Contra-indications Allergy or over-sensitivity to lemon

Skin damage or weeping, infected wounds on the lower legs

Material Basin, large enough to cover calves with water

1 organic lemon

Large and small towels

Procedure Pour water into the basin and add the lemon. Cut the lemon in the water and squeezed well, before removing it (for details, see page 69).

The recipient sits in a relaxed position for the footbath, with the upper legs and hips covered with a large towel to maintain warmth.

The feet are placed in the footbath for 5 to 10 minutes, or as long as the footbath is comfortable.

To enhance the effect, a soft blanket may be wrapped around the recipient's shoulders and allowed to fall to the floor encasing the footbath.

Rest 10 minutes.

Finishing off Dry the feet well with the small towel, and put on warm socks. Empty the footbath, wash and dry it.

Mustard (Brassica nigra)

Through increasing the metabolic activity in the feet one can ease increased metabolic processes in the head. With this application the recipient is better able to be conscious of the feet, which enables better incarnation.

In spite of the momentary aggressive nature of mustard, this can be very helpful before sleep. The legs may be oiled with lavender oil after the bath is completed.

Indications Inflammatory processes in head; for instance, runny nose resulting in dull, dazed head, or sinusitis

Headache with red, congested head; beginning migraine

Morning low in depressed people

For people who find it difficult to wake up, with dazed
    head, a cotton wool feeling in legs and cold feet

Unrest and fear

Fixed thought patterns

Problems going to sleep that are related to not being
    completely awake during the day, or not being able
    to 'let go' properly at night

Activate postpartum lochia discharge

Skin damage, weeping or infected skin illnesses on the **Contra-indication**
    legs

Redness not yet dissipated from a previous compress

Allergic reaction to mustard

Menstruation, as a mustard footbath can cause very
    heavy bleeding

Vein problems, like varicose veins or thrombophlebitis

Mustard powder: 200 ml for a large, 25-litre footbath **Material**
    tub, 100 ml for a 10-litre bucket (1 fl oz per US gal)

Footbath tub or a large laundry bucket with hot water,
    37–38°C (98–100°F); the tub needs to be deep
    enough for the water to come just under the knees

Large bath towel or a light blanket

Towel for drying

Bowl to wash legs afterwards

Oil, if required

Wooden spoon

Put the mustard powder into the tub, add hot water and **Preparation**
mix well, removing all lumps. Move the water for about
a minute in a lemniscates (figure-of-8) movement using
a large wooden spoon.

The person should be sitting comfortably, while hav- **Procedure**
ing the footbath. Use a large towel to cover the legs
from the tub right up to the hips to retain warmth
and protect against the mustard smell and possible eye
irritation.

Duration The duration is between 15 and 20 minutes, depending on the patient's experience and as decided with the practitioner.

The first therapy with mustard is usually shorter as burning often occurs surprisingly fast. If a patient is feeling afraid or unsure then it is better to stop the therapy. The subsequent treatment can be longer if the recipient is happy and the skin reaction from the previous therapy is no longer visible.

Finishing off Clean the feet over the tub using water at body temperature. It is important that mustard is not left between the toes as this could continue to irritate. The feet may appear red, as if they had a pair of red socks on them. Carefully dry both feet and apply a neutral oil (for instance, olive oil) or an essential oil, using a few slow strokes, before putting on socks and letting the recipient lie down for a rest.

Pour the mustard water into a sink or toilet with a large drainage pipe, as a small one can easily become blocked. Clean the tub well with soap and dry it.

Rest After a footbath a rest is required of about 10 to 20 minutes depending on the patient's situation.

Rosemary (Rosmarinus officinalis)

Rosemary, like lavender belongs to the aromatic, Labiatae family that grows best in the Mediterranean. Rosemary's soft violet coloured flowers grow between the needle-like, hard, contracted leaves. The flower and leaf hold the valuable etheric oils. Rosemary has a deeply warming, activating, awakening effect as well as the quality of stimulating the circulation. Rosemary strengthens the heart and circulation and can even increase the blood pressure. A rosemary footbath can be given 1–2°C (2–4°F) higher than body temperature. The treatment must be experienced as comfortable and pleasant, with additional warm water added as needed.

Morning tiredness **Indications**
Arterial circulatory disturbances
Headaches, dizziness, sense of being dazed, inability to
    wake properly (often related to a low blood pressure)
Prior to menstruation, when the flow seems arrested for
    some reason
Difficulty settling at night especially when caused by
    lack of physical or mental activity in the day or a
    disturbed day/night rhythm

Allergy or over-sensitivity to rosemary **Contra-indications**
Venous complications such as serious varicose veins or
    venous infections like thrombophlebitis
Skin damage or weeping, infected wounds on the legs
First day of menstruation, when rosemary can increase
    blood flow

Basin, large enough to cover calves with water **Material**
10–15 ml (2–3 tsp) bathmilk
Large towel

Place water in the basin and add the bathmilk. Mix the **Procedure**
bathmilk in with your hand using a rhythmic lemnis-
cate (figure-of-8) movement for about a minute to re-
enliven the water.
    The recipient sits in a relaxed position for the foot-
bath, with the upper legs and hips covered with a large
towel to maintain warmth.
    Place the feet in the footbath for 15 to 30 minutes, as
long as the footbath is experienced as comfortable.

15 minutes. **Rest**

Dry the feet well with the small towel, and put on warm **Finishing off**
socks. Empty the footbath, wash and dry it.

3

Cloths and Compresses

Beeswax

A cloth is impregnated with melted beeswax, warmed and placed on the recipient's body for over two hours. A beeswax cloth is 15 × 25 cm (6 × 10 in) and can be made in the clinic or home. Beeswax cloths are produced by a number of different manufacturers in Germany. In the therapeutic laboratory of the Ita Wegman Clinic plantago beeswax cloths that contain a plantago lanceolata additive are made for bronchial conditions. Plantago beeswax cloths have the added expectorant effect from the plantago.

Beeswax has a strong, warming strength and energy. The bees collect the warm, sugary nectar and pollen from flowers. These substances are absorbed into the bee then changed and released as sweat that forms a sweet smelling, malleable wax. Wax's warmth quality can be experienced in a burning beeswax candle. When applied externally, beeswax produces dry, soft, constant warmth that is relaxing, calming and soothing.

Indications

Bronchitis, with painful, dry coughing; especially when there is a sense of raw pain in the bronchi and trachea
Pseudo croup
Aching joints

Contra-indications

Skin damage or weeping, infected wounds in the area being treated

Material Plantago beeswax cloth or another prepared beeswax cloth

Outer cloth to hold beeswax cloth *in situ,* or a firm warming piece of clothing such as a woollen singlet for a child

Warm hot-waterbottle

Manufacturing You need a thin cotton cloth that is the appropriate size,
your own cloth beeswax candle or block, and a small plastic bag.

Melt the wax and drip it onto a cloth, ensuring the layer of wax is even and thin. You could even lay the cloth onto a hot-waterbottle so the wax remains thin and spreads readily into the cloth. Alternatively, the wax could be melted in a double boiler* and the thin cotton cloth dipped in and held briefly to cool.

Procedure The wax cloth is either left in the plastic bag or laid on grease-proof paper and warmed on a hot-waterbottle. The cloth needs to be a little warmer than body temperature and, depending on the hot-waterbottle temperature, may take 3 to 5 minutes to warm. Through warming, the wax becomes soft and pliable so that it moulds to the body form. Take the wax cloth out of the bag and apply it to the skin, securing it either with a binder or firm clothing.

Duration Apply for a number of hours, or even all night, for as long as it is experienced as comfortable.

Finishing off When removed, keep the skin warm and protected with warm clothing or a firm binder.

Return the beeswax cloth to the plastic bag and reuse until it becomes dry, cracked or loses its characteristic aroma.

---

* A pot inside a larger pot containing water, preventing the inner pot from boiling..

Bolus eucalyptus comp. *(Bolus alba compositum & Eucalyptus globulus)*

Bolus alba is manufactured at the Ita Wegman Clinic, Arlesheim. The base is a paste made from kaolinite (white earth or kaolin) and glycerine, with etheric oils of eucalyptus *(Eucalyptus globulus)*, rosemary *(Rosmarinus officinale)* and peppermint *(Metha piperita)* added. Eucalyptus comp. chest paste from Weleda can be used in a similar manner to the Bolus alba paste.

The paste is thick and it is spread on a cloth and used as a warmed poultice that is held in place with cotton and woollen binders for a number of hours.

This poultice has a warming, stimulating, anti-inflammatory and expectorant effect.

Chest, back, neck and breast compresses

Indications for chest and back compress

Chronic bronchitis with thick, slow moving mucus
Recuperating bronchitis & pneumonia
Asthma in children: to relieve difficult breathing rather than during the acute stage of an asthma attack
Post–pseudo croup attack: to relax and calm and as a follow–up treatment
This compress is often applied before sleep or when breathing difficulties develop

Indications for neck and throat compress

Painful throat infection
Glandular fever, when throat is involved
Acute stiff or bent neck
Swollen, infected parotid glands
This compress is often applied before sleep or when difficulties develop

Indications for breast compress

Hardened, inflamed and infected lymphatic breast tissue, when breast feeding
This compress can be applied a number of times daily depending on the situation.

Contra-indications Allergic reactions to any of the paste ingredients
Irritations due to open tissues or weeping, inflamed skin
in the area being treated

Material Bolus alba paste
Spatula
Inner cloth: a double layer fabric 2–3 cm (1 in) larger
than the area being treated
Outer cloth
Padding; clean woollen fleece or cotton combine, 2–3
cm (1 in) larger than the inner cloth
Warm hot-waterbottle
Plastic bag

Procedure Immediately before treatment prepare the paste cloth by
applying the paste 2–3 mm ($^1/_8$ in) thick on half the cloth,
leaving a 2–3 cm (1 in) edge. Fold the cloth together.
Warm the paste cloth on the hot-waterbottle with the
padding and outer cloth so it is warm when applied to
the body. The hot-waterbottle may be protected by using
a plastic bag when heating the paste cloth.

The paste cloth is applied in the prescribed area and
the warm padding applied on top to maintain warmth,
with the outer cloth wrapped and fastened securely.

Caution Do not overheat the paste, as the etheric oils will evaporate.

Duration The paste cloth can be applied for a number of hours
or throughout the night. It should be pleasantly warm,
without producing too much perspiration.

Finishing off After removing the paste cloth wash the skin and dry
as necessary. A thin cloth may be used as a wrap to
maintain warmth and protection for a number of hours
afterwards.

The paste cloth can be reused or disposed of as desired.
Clean and pack away the outer cloth and padding.

Rest 15 minutes, as needed

Calendula flower juice *(Calendula officinalis)*

Calendula grows profusely and abundantly. The flowers have a balanced and symmetrical form, while the leaf and stalk have a strong aromatic resin aroma. Calendula supports the healing of wounds through its anti–inflammatory qualities and by activating the body's natural life forces and self-cleansing.

Wound compress

Slow healing or superficially infected wounds such as **Indications** lower leg ulcer, bed sores and slow healing perineum following episiotomy

Open, bleeding or infected nipples of breast-feeding women, ideally cleansing nipples with calendula juice before breast feeding

This compress can be used a number of times in the day, depending on what is required.

Allergy to calendula **Contra-indications**

10 fresh, open calendula flowers **Material for juice**
Sharp knife & wooden chopping board
Mortar & pestle
Small bowl
Number large gauze dressings or pieces of muslin as required
Glass storage jar or bottle that has been rinsed with boiled water and has a well sealed lid

Combine dressing or gauze as required **Material for**
Outer cloth or elastic bandage as appropriate **wound dressing**
Disposable gloves if needed

Place the calendula flowers on a damp chopping board **Preparation of** to retain their juices. Cut the flowers finely, then placed **juice** in the mortar with a little fresh, cold water to cover the flowers. Grind the mixture with the pestle. Lay a dampened gauze dressing over the bowl, and pour the contents of the mortar onto it. Squeeze the gauze well to release the calendula juices. Reuse the plant remains by dipping in fresh water and squeezing again. Strain the final juice through gauze into the storage bottle. Note the preparation date on the bottle and store in the fridge.

Throw away the used gauze and flower leftovers. Wash and dry the utensils.

Freshly prepared calendula juice is a light golden yellow, becoming orange after a short while. The prepared juice can be used for 2 to 3 days if refrigerated.

Procedure Soak a gauze compress in the fresh juice and squeezed a little before placing over the wound. Use additional compresses to cover and secure the wound.

Normal awareness of hygiene is required. For infected wounds use disposable gloves.

Continue treatment as required.

Duration The compress is left on for 10 to 30 minutes.

Eucalyptus oil *(Eucalyptus globulus* 100%)

Eucalyptus or the fever tree is a tall fast-growing tree from Australia. It absorbs large quantities of water from wet ground, builds a hard wood and has thin tough leaves. The leaves contain much etheric oil and radiate a distinct aroma. The eucalyptus has a strong light and warmth quality.

Effect Through the intense warmth of the eucalyptus cloth the blood vessels widen, circulation increases, and there is a general relaxing and loosening in the area being treated. Through the initial warmth impulse caused by the hot inner compress, the warming effect of the oil can be established and continue undisturbed.

Eucalyptus oil has an antiseptic and anti-inflammatory effect.

Undiluted eucalyptus oil must not be taken internally or **Caution**
applied to exposed skin; it is toxic to the kidneys. Keep
away from children.

Bladder compress

Nervous bladder with frequent nocturnal micturition **Indications**
Acute and chronic bladder infections
Cystitis
This compress is usually given immediately before bed-
time and if there is a problem or need.

First day of menstruation as the hot application on the **Contra-indications**
  bladder region can stimulate heavy bleeding
Allergies or sensitivity to eucalyptus or the oil base
Skin damage where there are moist, inflamed or infected
  skin lesions in the area of the compress application.

5 drops pure eucalyptus oil **Material**
300 ml (10 fl oz) hot water at approximately 75°C
  (170°F)
Shallow bowl
Inner cloth
Wringing-cloth
Outer cotton binder and woollen binder (outer cloths
  need to be large enough to encompass the body)
Safety pins
Hot-waterbottle

For more details see *Liver, abdominal and kidney compresses* **Procedure**
on page 22.
    Fold the inner cloth to 15 × 20 cm (6 × 8 in). Roll
the outer cloth from the sides towards the middle and
pre-warm with a hot-waterbottle.
    Pour hot water in the bowl and add drops of eucalyp-
tus oil which quickly disperses across the surface.
    Roll out the outer cloths and lay them behind the
sitting patient who lies down on them.
    Lay the inner cloth flat on top of the water so water
and oil are equally absorbed. Lay the wringing-cloth

next to the bowl. Lay the inner cloth on it and wring them out well. Remove the inner cloth from the wringing-cloth and lay on the bladder as quickly as possible ensuring the side that has absorbed the oil is on the skin. Wrap the outer cloths are quickly and well wrapped around the patient. To ensure the wet inner cloth does not become cold it is especially important that the outer cloth is warm. No hot-waterbottles are needed.

Duration 20–30 minutes, or shorter if the compress is experienced as cold

Finishing off Remove cloths. Rinse the inner cloth in warm water and wring out. Hang to dry with the outer cloths.

Rest Quarter to half hour

Kidney compress

Indications Acute and chronic bladder infections
Cystitis, pyelitis
This compress is usually given immediately before bedtime and if there is a problem or need.

Contra-indications First day of menstruation as the hot application on the kidney region can stimulate heavy bleeding
Allergies or sensitivity to eucalyptus or the oil base
Skin damage where there are moist, inflamed or infected skin lesions in the area of the compress application

Material 5 drops pure eucalyptus oil
300 ml (10 fl oz) hot water approximately 75°C (170°F)
Shallow bowl
Inner cloth
Wringing-cloth
Outer cotton binder and woollen binder (outer cloths need to be large enough to encompass the torso)
Safety pins
Hot-waterbottle

For more details see *Liver, abdominal and kidney compresses* **Procedure** on page 22.

Fold the inner cloth to 15 × 20 cm (6 × 8 in). Roll the outer cloth from the sides towards the middle and pre-warm with a hot-waterbottle.

Pour hot water in the bowl and add drops of eucalyptus oil which quickly disperses across the surface.

Roll out the outer cloths and lay them behind the sitting patient who lies down on them.

Lay the inner cloth flat on top of the water so water and oil are equally absorbed. Lay the wringing-cloth next to the bowl. Lay the inner cloth on it and wring them out well. Remove the inner cloth from the wringing-cloth and lay on the kidneys as quickly as possible ensuring the side that has absorbed the oil is on the skin. Wrap the outer cloths are quickly and well wrapped around the patient. To ensure the wet inner cloth does not become cold it is especially important that the outer cloth is warm. No hot-waterbottles are needed.

20–30 minutes, or shorter if the compress is experi- **Duration** enced as cold

Remove cloths. Rinse the inner cloth in warm water **Finishing off** and wring out. Hang to dry with the outer cloths.

Quarter to half hour   **Rest**

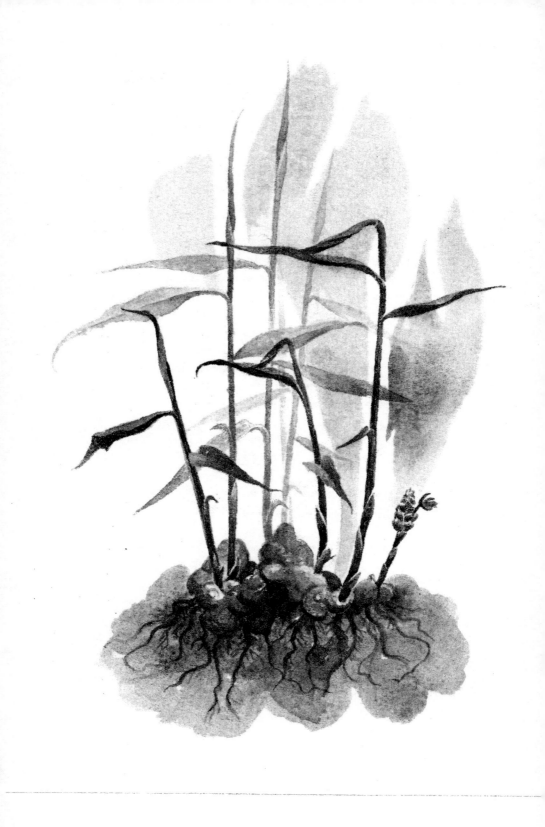

Ginger *(Zingiber officinale)*

Ginger thrives in warm, damp, tropical conditions. Between the ginger root and stem is a rhizome that lies flat on the earth. From the rhizome roots develop, divide and multiply. Ginger is quick growing, with thin shoots up to a metre (3 ft) high, lance type leaves and separate flower stems. The flower stem thickens at the tip like the ears of a corn plant to protect the orchid like flower that opens in the evening. The tongue of the flower is pale yellow, with purple spots. Each flower only lives for one blooming and is spent the following day. The leaf stem develops horizontal leaves that have a clear, ordered structure. The leaves are dark green and buried under them lie the flower stalks, with the secretive flowers that can only be seen at dusk.

The rhizome is harvested, when the flowers have withered. The fresh rhizome is hard and juicy, and smells fresh and spicy, almost citrus like. The ginger juice is aromatic, with a sharp and spicy taste. The leaves and flower stems have similar smelling and tasting juices. While the whole plant contains etheric oil, the oil is primarily in the rhizome. Ginger has an intense but mild seasoning strength, which stimulates the digestive system. People with a delicate digestion find it quite acceptable.

Effect The tropical sun does not result in large coloured flowers; rather the power of the sun has been internalised into the whole plant, especially the rhizome. The fire of the plant has been contained into an inward glowing ember, with a long lasting glimmer present in the rhizome.

When ginger is taken into the body, gentle, long-lasting warmth is generated from within that glows and spreads widely. Because of this effect, chronic inflammations can be activated and healed, hardening and stagnation can be loosened, and organs stimulated.

Neutral oil, such as almond or olive oil, may be used after the compress to maintain inner warmth.

Dry ginger powder is used in the compress preparation.

The expected warmth comes 5 to 10 minutes after the compress has been applied on the body. Before this, the patient can feel cool and uncomfortable. Hot-waterbottles can be used on the patient's sides or feet. Once the compress is working, they can be taken away so the warmth process continues without being disturbed by the additional outer warmth. The ability of the patient finding their own inner warmth increases with the number of applications.

During the ginger compress treatment, including the rest, many people sleep while others enter a dreamy state often with intensive, imaginative experiences. When the treatment is complete and the recipient fully awake, there is often increased alertness and eagerness to be active.

CAUTION Occasionally, ginger cannot be used because of the allergic response and an inability to cope with ginger. For some people there is a slight, allergic skin irritation. Sometimes the ginger compress can also cause nausea and circulatory problems; care needs to be taken with hypertensive patients. Disturbing or threatening memories of the past can also occur.

Using less ginger can diminish the uncomfortable reaction, sense of burning or intense reddening. Alternatively, the compress cloth can be squeezed within a tea towel so less ginger is on the cloth reducing the effect.

Kidney compress

The enlivened functioning within the kidneys rays to the whole organism. There seems to be a relationship between this raying out and the soul of the patient, between how the soul relates to the organism.

Indications Constitutional conditions such as unsettled, agitated, or overactive mental processes
Low blood pressure and vegetative disturbances
Arthritis conditions such as osteoarthritis and rheumatoid arthritis

Weak metabolic processes as found with irritable bowel
   syndrome and anorexia nervosa
Patients slow to be active in the mornings (following
   the compress, they feel really awake and active)

An intolerance to ginger, allergic response **Contra-indications**
The commencement of menstruation because men-
   strual flow can be loosened and activated too quickly
Where there are weeping, infected skin lesions in the
   area of the compress application

1 heaped teaspoon ginger powder **Material**
500 ml (17 fl oz) water at 75°C (170°F)
Shallow bowl
Compress cloth
Cotton binder and woollen binder to hold the compress
   on firmly (needs to be 4 or 5 times larger than the
   compress cloth)
Safety pins
Two hot–waterbottles, if necessary
Face-cloth
Neutral oil, like almond or olive oil

This compress is done early in the morning, sometimes **Procedure**
before rising. If the recipient seems unsettled during the
compress, then the rest time can be shortened and the
person activated earlier.
   In chronic conditions the compress may be applied
daily for at least seven consecutive days for maximum
effect.
   Prepare the binders; roll out to fit the back. Prepare
the ginger and hot water in a bowl mix this well.
   Place the compress cloth in the water so the surface
of the cloth is evenly covered with the ginger, lay this on
the wringing-cloth and wring well (the drier the cloth
the warmer it stays).
   Place the compress cloth on the inner binder and
position this on the part of the body being treated,
ensuring the compress cloth is comfortably warm and
positioned well. Wrap the patient with the woollen

binder and hold in place with the pins. Add hot-water-bottles to each side and the feet if the patient feels cool. If there is scoliosis (hollow back) place a small cushion in the back.

Chest and back compresses

The deep and intensive warmth activates stagnant, hardened processes in the lungs. The viscous mucus can be loosened, relieving the lungs.

Indications Final stages of pneumonia or bronchitis
Cold, sub-febrile pneumonia especially when antibiotics have been given and the fever has been reduced artificially.

Contra-indications An intolerance to ginger, allergic response
The commencement of menstruation because menstrual flow can be loosened and activated too quickly
Where there are weeping, infected skin lesions in the area of the compress application

Material As for *Kidney compress* above.

Preparation Generally, these applications are done in the morning.
In order to establish a good effect with the chest application, often the back and chest application are applied at the same time, using two cloths rather than one.
Fold and prepare the binders with a hot-waterbottle warming them. The compress cloth is 40 × 120 cm (16 × 48 in) and can be folded three times to 20 × 30 cm (8 × 12 in), thus becoming smaller and thicker. Place the compress cloth in the wringer cloth as necessary.

Procedure for back compress Prepare the binders; roll out to fit the back. Prepare the ginger and hot water in a bowl mix this well.
Place the compress cloth in the water so the surface of the cloth is evenly covered with the ginger, lay this on the wringing-cloth and wring well.

Place the compress cloth on the inner binder and position this on the part of the body being treated, ensuring the compress cloth is comfortably warm and positioned well. Wrap the patient with the woollen binder and hold in place with the pins. Add hot-water-bottles to each side and the feet if the patient feels cool. If there is scoliosis (hollow back) place a small cushion in the back.

Prepare two binders, for the patient to lie on. Prepare the ginger and hot water as above and put the compress cloth in the bowl, wring well. **Procedure for chest compress**

Lay the compress cloth on the chest ensuring it is positioned so the ginger is on the skin. Pin the binders firmly

Use hot-waterbottles only if necessary

30 to 40 minutes, depending on the desired intensity. Remove the compress earlier if it cools, or if the patient has an itching or burning sensation. **Duration**

It is important not to disturb the patient in this time. If the patient enters into a heavy, dark state after the compress or has difficulty waking then a shorter treatment is advisable.

Remove cloths. Wash the body with water at body temperature, as any ginger powder left may disturb the skin. Dry well. Apply the oil using quiet movements in order that the warmth is retained. This stage is optional. **Finishing off**

Afterwards wrap the patient in a fresh, warm cloth so they can rest for 20 to 30 minutes. This wrapping-cloth is light, soft and warm (such as molleton) to avoid speedy cooling.

It is best for the patient not to fall asleep during the treatment as they may have difficulty waking. It is also important not to disturb the patient during rest time. If the patient is restless or unsettled, then shorten the rest to 5 or 10 minutes.

Afterwards they should get up and be active.

Healing clay

There are a number of different types of healing clay depending on the origin that influences the substances contained in the clay. Generally healing clay has a high percentage of silica and other minerals.

Healing clay is mixed with water to a thick paste and spread on a cloth as a poultice. It is applied moist and either warm or cool and left applied to the skin to evaporate naturally until the clay becomes dry. Depending on the condition and the desired therapeutic effect a lotion (such as arnica or meadowsweet) or herb tea may be added.

Effect Healing clay is used for conditions of congestion and inflammation in the body. It is able to bring structure and movement through silica's strong forming qualities. The clay's silica structure is able to bring back a healthy form and draw out bacteria and metabolic waste products that cause illness in the body. The resulting evaporation of the clay that occurs while the poultice is applied has an analgesic and natural detoxification effect both internally and externally.

CAUTION The skin in the area being treated needs to always be warm so the healing clay can dry out and evaporate. If the healing clay feels cold or excessively cooling then it needs to be removed. The clay must not be mixed in a metal bowl (like copper, cast iron or aluminium) that may oxidise changing the clay's healing qualities.

Indications Swollen joints such as arthritis
Insect bites, abscesses and furuncles
Thrombophlebitis
Throat infection with painful swallowing especially
    when a cooling compress on the neck is beneficial
Infected or weeping wounds such as a leg ulcer

Contra-indications None

1 tsp healing clay in warm or cold water **Material**
Small (ceramic) mixing bowl
Inner cloth, double layered, 2–3 cm (1 in) larger than
  the area being treated
several large pieces of gauze
Hot–waterbottle in a protective plastic bag
Bed protection as appropriate
Outer cloth or elastic bandage
Face–cloth to clean the area after the treatment
Neutral oil such as olive or almond oil

The healing clay and water are mixed in the bowl to **Preparation**
form a spreadable paste. Dampen the inner cloth to avoid
the clay drying out too quickly. Spread the paste 3–5 mm
($^{1}/_{8}$ in) thick on the inner cloth leaving an edge free on all
sides. Cover the clay with a piece of gauze so that it does
not adhere to the skin, and is easier to remove.

   People who are sensitive to the cold find the clay cloth
more comfortable when warmed on a hot–waterbottle
(cover the bottle with a plastic bag for protection).

   Cover the bed with a protector and place the outer
cloth under the area to be treated.

Place the clay poultice on the recipient's skin with the **Procedure**
gauze side on the skin. Wrap the outer cloth firmly
around the body and secure. An additional bandage may
be used (for instance, on a joint) to avoid the clay crum-
bling and spilling out. Leave the poultice on for 1 to 2
hours. The clay is generally dry after this time.

Following removal of the poultice, clean the skin with **Finishing off**
lukewarm water and dry well. If the recipient experi-
ences a sense of dryness on the skin after the treatment
then apply a neutral oil. Either disposed of the inner
cloth or wash it with warm water for reuse.

   Empty and, if necessary, clean the hot–waterbottles.
Clean all wrapping–cloths, dry and leave to air

Quarter to half hour **Rest time**

Honey

A natural, good quality honey that is neither too thin nor hard is used for this treatment. The honey is spread on a cotton cloth and applied for a number of hours. The honey that we use for wound treatments is sometimes so runny that we have to apply it with a syringe.

Effect Honey has a special connection to the quality of warmth. The bees collect pollen and nectar, transform and store it in the warmth of the hive. Honey provides a deeply warming effect that relaxes irritated and overly stimulated and sensitive areas of the body. Honey conveys a special structural forming energy — related to the six sided hexagon structure of the honeycomb — that has anti-bacterial, anti-inflammatory and cleansing qualities. Bees keep their hive at a constant temperature of 36°C (97°F), similar to the human body's.

CAUTION If a honey treatment is applied to a diabetic person, it can cause hyperglycemia.

Compresses for bronchitis, neck and wounds

Indications Bronchitis with a painful, irritating cough
Sore throat with pain on swallowing and irritation in the throat
Infected wounds such as lower leg and decubitus ulcers

Contra-indications Diabetes
Allergy to honey

Material Honey and spatula
Inner cloth double layered, 2–3 cm (1 in) larger than the application area
Gauze if necessary
Outer cloth with elastic bandages if necessary
Hot-waterbottle, with protective plastic bag

Spread the honey thinly over the inner cloth and lay a **Preparation**
piece of gauze on top leaving an edge around the inner
cloth. For sensitive parts of the body warm the honey to
body temperature using the hot–waterbottle.

Apply the honey cloth to the appropriate part of the **Procedure**
body and secure firmly. Depending on the type of
wound and its size, the honey can be applied directly
into the wound area either using a syringe or a spatula.
It is especially important that the honey only covers the
actual wound and not the edges of the wound.

   Apply the honey cloth for one or more hours. When
removed, the honey should be completely absorbed by
the skin.

   If some pieces of gauze are left on the skin they can
be washed away with lukewarm water.

When the compress is removed, the skin can be **Finishing off**
washed with lukewarm water and dried if a little sticky.
Following treatment, cover the area and protect from
cold or draughts.

   Dispose of the honey cloth, clean the hot–waterbottle.

Quarter hour   **Rest time**

Horseradish *(Cochlearia armoracia)*

Horseradish is a plant with strong vitality. Over a number of years it develops a large strong root and tough leaves, with many small inconspicuous flowers. In this plant fiery-hot sulfurous oils have been stored in the root. The root contains an extraordinary hot vitality.

Horseradish, like mustard, belongs to the Cruciferae family and contains a substance known as Allyl isothio-cyanate oil,. This oil is colourless, with a pungent taste similar to mustard. Allyl isothiocyanate oil is typical of the Cruciferae family and in large amounts is extremely irritating to the skin. This oil creates a local artificial inflammation causing the skin to redden and feel as if it is burning. When applied on the skin for too long horseradish may cause the skin to blister and burn.

Horseradish root is freshly grated and placed in a thin cotton cloth that is folded and sealed then applied for a short period of time. If fresh horseradish is unavailable, grated horseradish without preservatives can be used. Freshly grated garlic can also be used as an alternative. For those requiring a follow-up treatment or with very sensitive skin, horseradish ointment can used.

CAUTION The recipient needs to be well informed about this treatment in order to be prepared for the initial painful and hot effect. Often following the treatment, a real sense of relieve is experienced. Horseradish treatments require the practitioner to be aware and observant, providing good support to the recipient in order that the appropriate duration for the treatment is provided. During this treatment, stay with the recipient, especially for the first time.

Prepare horseradish treatment carefully as even the aroma can irritate the mucus membranes of the eyes. During an application, the recipient's eyes need to be closed and the practitioner's hands well washed after contact with the grated root. The recipient's skin is usually red after the treatment. After 24 hours this reddening should have receded and disappeared. If the skin is over-irritated neutral oil such as almond or olive oil can be applied. If intensive burning occurs it is treated like a sunburn with Weleda combudoron cream or similar.

If horseradish is applied regularly or in special cases the skin overreacts and becomes irritated, itchy, burnt or blistered then the treatment needs to stop. Skin sensitivity can vary between people depending on the skin type, for example people with blonde or red hair who react strongly to sunlight, often react very intensely.

Compresses on the forehead, neck and nasal passages

Chronic inflammation of forehead and nasal passages **Indications**
    such as sinusitis
Headache or beginning of migraine, when a neck compress may be used

Allergy to horseradish   **Contra-indication**
Damaged, weeping skin in the area of the compress
Past redness from a previous horseradish application

Horseradish root   **Material**
Knife and fine grater
Plastic gloves
Gauze compress or thin cloth with tape
Face-cloth, gauze or cloth to place over the compress to protect the skin and eyes
Vaseline, if necessary

Lay out a thin cloth or gauze for the compress. Put on **Preparation** plastic gloves and clean the horseradish root, and grate it over the compress. Grate enough to cover half the cloth with a layer 1 cm ($\frac{1}{2}$ in) thick, fold the other half over and tape down well to form a neat package. If the grated root is too dry and rubbery, add a little water.

Hold the horseradish compress to the area without any **Procedure** pressure. If the recipient is able to keep their eyes closed during the entire treatment, they can hold the compress and regulate the pressure and duration themselves. If this is not possible, the practitioner holds the compress and the recipient holds a dampened or dry face-cloth over their eyes.

For restless people or children, protect the eyes with Vaseline and small cotton squares. After the treatment, remove the Vaseline with a dry cloth.

Duration Leave on for no longer than 1 to 3 minutes. The recipient can decide the length of time for each treatment. The duration is affected by the quality and freshness of the horseradish root.

Finishing off Dispose of the horseradish compress. Wash the face-cloths and outer cloths with warm water and hang out to dry.

Rest time Quarter to half hour

Lemon *(Citrus limonum)*

When a lemon is cut the aroma stimulates salivation. The refreshing lemon oil is used as an additive in pot-pourris, cosmetics, confectionary and drinks. In order for the aromatic qualities to develop, lemons require considerable light and warmth in their development. The lemon tree grows to a height of up to 7 metres (23 ft). It has leaves, flowers and fruit throughout the entire year. The thorny branches are thickly covered by simple, leather-like, tough leaves, which when rubbed release an aromatic smell. From the white, bewitching, sweet-smelling flower the fruit ripens within half a year, producing a hard, round, juicy fruit. Unlike most subtropical fruits the citrus fruits do not have a soft, watery flesh. Rather the juice is in elongated cells lying closely together. The cells are enclosed in a membrane forming the characteristic radial segments. The lemon's leathery, tough skin prevents the flesh drying out.

A lemon always remains sour. Despite the intensive sun, it remains sour when ripe, unlike other fruits which produce sugar in ripening. The fruit falls from the tree in this 'unripe state' and remains juicy for a long time without becoming overripe or rotten. The lemon juice contains various fruit acids, fruit sugar, vitamin C and potassium.

Beside the fleeting presence of the aromatic scent of the flowers, the lemon fruit displays a drawing-in tendency, an inwardly directed movement. This is reflected in the development of the fruit cells that grow from the skin into the middle of the fruit. The abundant etheric oil is in the oil sacs in the large pores of the skin. This oil is only released when the skin is cut. This pent-up energy of the oil is also seen in the un-ripening tendency of the fruit.

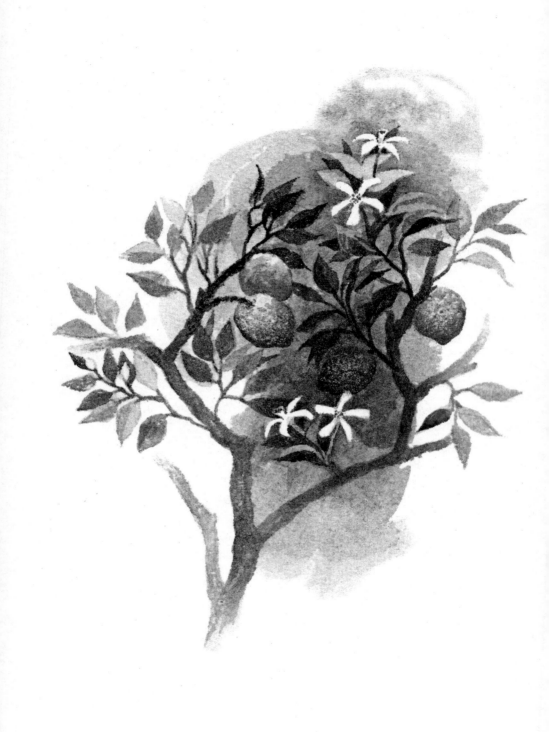

The lemon works through its intense sour, drawing- **Effect**
in effect that stimulates salivation, contracts tissue and
refreshes. Lemon etheric oils have an antibacterial, anti-
inflammatory effect and the fresh fruity smell of lemon
oil is awakening and enlivening.

In the lemon there is an especially restrained energy
working 'from the outer to the inner.'[1] It is through
this quality the lemon has a structuring tendency
that restrains overactive metabolic processes caused by
inflammation or an unformed or congested watery
(etheric) organism.

A lemon application can irritate the skin and is not **CAUTION**
tolerated by all people. In the case of an allergic rash or
burning, the treatment must be stopped.

Wash an organic lemon under hot water to remove dirt **Preparation of**
or wax prior to use.   **lemon water**

Fill a bowl with water
and place the lemon in the
water. Cut in half using a
sharp knife and pierce the
skin a number of times to
release and disperse the etheric oils.

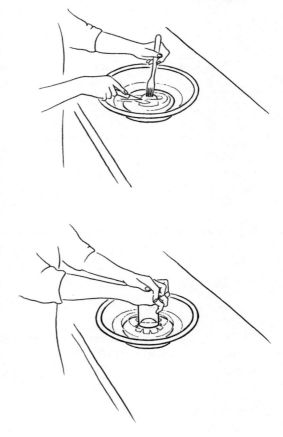

Cut the lemon in a star-
like form from the outside
inwards, and then press to
release the juice under the
water. If using very hot
water, you can hold the
lemon is place with a fork
and press with a glass.

If no organic lemon is
available, then use the juice
of half a lemon.

Because the etheric oils
disperse quickly, it is important that lemon water is
prepared immediately prior

to use. Ideally, prepare the water near the patient so they can breathe in the etheric oils from the surrounding air.

For fever reducing calf compresses, an alternative can be used such as apple cider vinegar.

A citrus bathmilk is not a substitute for a fresh lemon as during manufacture soap is used to create the emulsion.

Chest compress

Ideally, this hot chest compress is applied with two people due to the size and relatively thin fabric used for the inner cloth. The compress can cool quickly and the outer cloth needs to be wrapped around as quickly as possible. Good preparation and rapid application are very important.

This compress has a heat releasing effect. The forming and structuring quality of the lemon reduces inflammatory, infectious processes in the lung connected with excess water and mucus production.

Indications Chest infections such as pneumonia and bronchitis
This compress is often used for patients with a high fever. For this reason no hot-waterbottles are used.

Caution Observe the recipient carefully during the compress for any sign of discomfort, avoiding perspiring, chilling, restriction or pressure. Often after the compress, the person is tired and needs to sleep.

Contra-indications Allergy to lemon; skin infections or weeping wounds or cuts in the application area

Material One organic lemon
$^1/_2$ litre ($^1/_2$ quart) very hot water (70–80°C, 160–175°F)
Knife, fork, glass
Inner compress and wringing-cloth
Outer cloth that is large enough to encompass the entire upper chest region

Fold the inner cloth to the correct width and roll the **Procedure**
ends towards the middle. Then roll the wringing-cloth
around it. Similarly roll the outer cloth from the ends
towards the middle and warm with a hot-waterbottle.
(For a full description see *Body and chest compress,*
page 26.)

Prepare the lemon water (see page 69).

Place the outer cloth behind the back of the recipient. Put the inner cloth in the lemon water, soak well
and wring out until no moisture is left. Take the inner
cloth out of the wringing-cloth, roll out across the
back and apply as hot as possible. Wrap the outer cloth
around promptly. The recipient lies back on the bed.

If two people are applying the compress, they stand
to the right and left of the recipient. They roll the inner
cloth out at the same time, applying it as hot as possible over the flanks and chest, rapidly securing with the
outer cloth.

If only one person is applying the compress, they roll
one side fully out wrapping around as hot as possible
and immediately covering with the outer cloth then
they continue with the other side. The outer cloth is
firmly secured.

If hot-waterbottles are required, they are only used to
maintain body warmth on the flanks and not placed on
the chest, which could restrict the breathing or cause
heat to go to the head.

Half to three-quarters of an hour **Duration**

Remove the cloths. Rinse the inner cloth and hang out **Finishing off**
to dry with the outer cloth.

Quarter to half an hour **Rest time**

Calf compress

The inner cloths are soaked in lemon water, 2–3°C (4–5°F) below the recipient's body temperature. They are wrapped around the feet and calves up to the knees. The outer cloths are wrapped over the inner cloth and secured firmly. As a sudden drop in temperature is taxing and can cause the temperature to rise again, wool cloths are used for the outer cloths.

Effect Through this cooling compress, a release of body warmth is achieved. The goal is not to achieve a sudden drastic drop in body temperature; rather it is enough to reduce the temperature by 1–2°C (2–4°F). This reduces the peak of the temperature so the recipient copes more comfortably with the fever. The lemon has an ordering effect on the recipient's congested fluid organism, which can be seen in the perspiring face during the fever. Lemon is also refreshing and anti-bacterial.

Indications Lemon calf compresses are given when there is a high fever, with headaches causing agitation and disturbance, even hallucinating. An individual may be disturbed with a temperature as low as 38°C or as high as 40°C (100.5–104°F), so it is important to consider each case as unique. Generally, rises in body temperatures have a beneficial effect on the metabolism and assist in countering the negative effects of infections. It is for this reason that calf compresses are only used when there is concern for the wellbeing of the individual, and usually after discussion with the physician.

CAUTION Calf compresses must not be applied if the feet are cold. This would cause the fever to become further centralized without warmth being transferred out of the body through the legs. In this case first warm the feet using a hot-waterbottle, footbath or oiling. Through this the warmth is more readily dispersed throughout the body and often this is enough to reduce the body temperature.

During the treatment observe the recipient closely for perspiring, changes in colour of the face and in consciousness. If the situation does not settle and the fever continues to increase, a different treatment or medication for decreasing the temperature may need to be given. Depending on the situation and how the recipient responds, an assistant may be required to hold the leg when the lemon compress is being applied.

Contra-indications

Allergy to lemon

Skin infections or weeping wounds or cuts in the application area

Material

1 lemon

500–750 ml (17–25 fl oz) water (2–3°C, 2–4°F below body temperature)

Shallow bowl

Sharp knife

4 inner cloths or cotton bandages (for children cotton socks may be used)

2 outer cloths (for children large woollen socks may be used)

Bed protection

Procedure

Fold all inner cloths to a width of 15–20 cm (6–8 in) and roll up. Also roll up the outer cloths.

Prepare lemon water (see page 69).

Place bed protection under the legs. Place the inner cloths in the lemon water and wring out well. Wrap the first leg from the toes to the knee. Wrap the outer cloth immediately as the inner cloth is relatively thin and cools quickly. It is important to avoid gaps and folds in the fabric as the air pockets will act as a cooling agent. The outer cloths need to be applied flat with no thick folds as they may press on the skin and be uncomfortable.

A description for wrapping cloths around the legs is on pages 112f.

Cover the legs with a thin blanket. After 10 to 15

minutes remove the cloths. The inner cloths are usually dry by this time.

If necessary, add more water or even another half lemon to the lemon water. Dip another inner cloth into the lemon water, wring out, and wrap around the leg as before. Depending on the situation, the calf compresses can be repeated three times.

Duration About 1 hour.

If the recipient falls asleep during the treatment this is a good indication the calf compresses have achieved the required effect. The recipient is left to sleep even with the compresses on the legs.

Finishing off Tidy away the cloths and bed protection; rinse all cloths and air to dry.

Throat lemon compress

The throat compress relieves inflammatory conditions of the throat. A compress is either as hot as possible or cold. The effect depends on the symptoms; a cold compress relieves heat and swelling, while a hot compress is relaxing and relieves discomfort. The patient is often able to explain from experience whether a hot or cold compress is suitable.

Indications for a hot compress Throat infection with burning and pain when swallowing, for example, tonsillitis, pharyngitis and laryngitis
The beginning stages of a throat infection, with an irritated throat

Indications for a cold compress A throat infection with pain on swallowing, or extreme swelling, for example, tonsillitis or glandular fever

Contra-indications A lemon allergy
Skin infections, weeping wounds or cuts in the application area

Half a lemon **Material**
300 ml (10 fl oz) water, cold or hot
Shallow bowl
Sharp knife
Inner cloth about 90 cm (36 in) long
Outer cloth about 15–20 cm (6–8 in) wide and 100–
    150 cm (3–5 ft) long
Fork, glass
Wringing-cloth for hot compresses

There is a full description under *Body and chest compress,* **Procedure**
page 26.
    Fold the inner cloth to a width of about 10 cm (4 in)
and roll up. For a hot compress place the rolled inner
cloth in a wringing-cloth.
    Prepare lemon water (see page 69).
    Soak the inner cloth in the lemon water and wring
out well. Then quickly wrap around the throat. Wrap
the outer cloth around the inner cloth, avoiding any air
pockets, and fastened securely.

Half to three quarters of an hour, or as long as the **Duration**
patient is comfortable.

After the compress cover the throat with a silk or thin **Finishing off**
woollen scarf to maintain warmth and comfort.
    Remove the compress cloths. Wash the inner cloth
with warm water and hang to dry with the outer cloth.

Quarter to half an hour **Rest time**

Throat compress using lemon slices

For this compress, lemon slices are wrapped in a thin folded cotton cloth for a number of hours This compress reduces inflammation and is pleasantly cooling

Indications Throat infection with pain on swallowing, burning and extreme swelling

Contra-indications Allergy to lemon

Skin infections or weeping wounds or cuts in the application area

CAUTION This application is especially skin irritating so caution is required if left on for long periods.

Material 1 lemon

Sharp knife and chopping board

Inner cloth, about 20 × 60 cm (8 × 24 in)

Outer cloth about 20 × 90 cm (8 × 36 in)

Procedure Cut the lemon into $\frac{1}{2}$ cm ($\frac{1}{4}$ in) slices and place them in a row along the middle of the cotton cloth.

Fold the inner cloth to create a tidy package and with the heel of your hand press on the slices of lemon to release the lemon juices onto the cotton cloth.

Unroll the outer cloth. Lay the inner cloth with lemon slices on the throat, wrap the outer cloth around, and secure firmly.

Duration An hour or longer. The compress should feel comfortable. If not, remove it.

Finishing off After removing the compress, clean the throat with warm water and cover for 1 to 2 hours with a thin scarf to protect from the cold.

Throw away the lemon slices. Wash the inner cloth with warm water, and hang all cloths to dry.

Rest time Quarter to half an hour.

Linseed *(Linum usitatissimum)*

The seed from linseed or common flax is boiled in water until a thick consistency like porridge develops. This is spread on a cloth and applied as a hot poultice for a number of hours. Ideally, grind the seeds freshly (that can be ground in an electric coffee grinder). If whole seeds are used, they need to be cooked for an extended period of time until they have a thick consistency like porridge.

Effect Linseed contains a high percentage of fatty oils that give a strong warmth quality. A linseed poultice provides a gentle, enduring and deeply warming effect. Once heated, it retains warmth for a number of hours.

The seeds from fenugreek *(Trigonella foenum-graecum)* also can be instead, and they have a similar effect. Fenugreek contains slightly less fatty oil than linseed, with an additional silica component. Fenugreek seeds are always used whole (not ground). The preparation and method is the same as for the linseed.

Compress on the forehead and nasal passages

Indications Chronic inflammation of the sinuses in the forehead and the back of the nose (linseed may be used in combination with horseradish that has a more aggressive effect; they can be alternated over the nose, which relieves the skin and surrounding tissues)

Chronic inflammation of the middle ear (otitis media); this compress is applied from the temple, around the ear to the hairline

Pain caused by bone metastases

Back pain from tense, strained muscles, such as lumbago

Tension or spasm in the neck muscle, such as torticollis that can be congenital, acquired or spasmodic

Furuncle activation and stimulation; to bring more rapidly to a dissolving, discharging and healing

Inflammation of the nail bed such as paronychia

Contra-indication Skin damage or weeping in the area of the compress

Material Linseed: 5 tbsp for 10 × 10 cm (4 × 4 in) poultice
Water: 10 tbsp
Pot and wooden spoon
Large piece gauze or thin cotton and plaster (band–aid)
Hot–waterbottle in plastic bag
Outer cloth and bandage, as required
Wrapping–cloth or warmed clothing
Padding of cotton wool or wool wrapped in gauze 2–3 cm (1 in) larger than the compress

Preparation Place wool in the gauze or thin cloth and hold together as a package, then heat on a hot–waterbottle.
   Add 5 tbsp seeds to 10 tbsp water and slowly simmer until it reaches a thick sticky, viscous consistency like porridge. With ground seeds this takes 2 to 5 minutes. Stir the mixture continuously to avoid burning. Spread the hot porridge about 1 cm ($^1/_2$ in) thick on the thin cotton or gauze cloth. Fold the edges inwards to form an enclosed package and seal with plaster (band–aid). The poultice is kept warm on the hot–waterbottle covered in the plastic bag.

CAUTION A freshly prepared poultice can be very hot so the temperature must be tested on the lower arm prior to being applied.

Procedure The poultice is applied as hot as possible with the padding over it to maintain warmth for as long as possible. The outer cloth is wrapped around and fastened securely.

Duration 1 hour or longer, as long as it is experienced as warm, pleasant and beneficial.

Finishing off After removal of the poultice and padding, wrap the treated area to maintain the warmth.
   Dispose of the poultice. Clean the cloths and hang out to dry and air. Empty and clean the hot–waterbottle.

Rest time Quarter to half an hour

Mustard *(Brassica nigra)*

Black mustard is very similar to its close relation white mustard (*Sinapis alba*), which is far more common. Comparing these two plants, particular characteristics become apparent.

Both are old cultured plants, which are still grown today for their oils, flavour, use as animal feed and cover crop. As with many other hybrids they have vitality and a strong flowering impulse. Mustard is a fast growing plant producing small yellow flowers on many side branches. While still in buds the flowers seem compressed as if in a nest, while underneath round seeds ripen in long pods. Mustard grows especially well in light warm places and often in the wild along road edges and footpaths.

Black mustard grows more slowly, it is a bigger plant with stronger branches and darker leaves, which can be slightly blue coloured. The flowers of black mustard are a darker more intense yellow than that of the sulfur yellow of white mustard flowers. In general, black mustard is greener, juicy and more robust looking than white mustard, which dries out and looks burnt after its quick intensive flowering process.

The seeds of the black mustard are smaller and are covered in a dark brown shell. This causes the brown speckles in the yellow mustard powder when ground. White mustard powder is simply yellow.

The seeds of both plants show their fiery strength, when chewed. White mustard seeds are hot for a short time. Black mustard seeds, on the other hand, unfold their spicy-hot taste more slowly, but leave a longer lasting hot sensation in the mouth. Black mustard seeds contain a higher amount of glucosinolate (or mustard oil glycoside), and are therefore preferred for medicinal uses. White mustard is more often used for the production of table mustard due to its high fatty oil content.

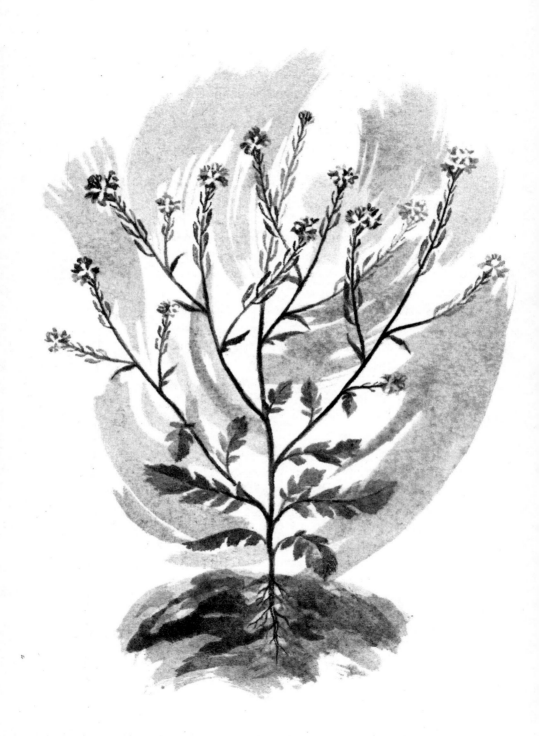

The mustard plant contains mustard oil which acts as a **Effect**
strong skin irritant and causes a local 'artificially induced
inflammation'. This can even become a burn on sensitive skin types if a compress is left on too long.

Increased circulation in the compress area shows that
the metabolic process becomes more active. This can
enable a diversion of the infection from within the body
towards the skin.

One can also look at these phenomena in another
way, and see that, through the increased experience of
pain (burning) and the increased blood flow (warmth
on the skin), the body becomes more aware and awake.
This can be called an incarnating effect, with the astral
and ego bodies drawing closer to the physical body.
The astral and ego are associated with pain and warmth
respectively.

In spite of the rather aggressive and momentary
effects of the mustard application, it is a very good
evening therapy.

In most cases the burning sensation of the skin begins **Typical pattern of**
surprisingly fast, reaching the first climax in only a few **burning sensation**
minutes. The sensation then becomes less and remains
fairly constant; this phase is often experienced as pleasant. Afterwards the burning increases again, eventually
becoming unbearable; the therapy is completed before
this second climax becomes intolerable.

After taking off the compress the burning sensation
continues, lessening only gradually. After a few minutes or possibly hours the burning sensation usually
decreases. In rare cases it can increase over this period
and in some very rare cases the skin may become even
redder hours after the therapy.

If the purpose of the compress is to warm and at the **Oil application**
same time to stimulate an organ region, neutral oil is
applied on the skin upon the completion of the compress. The after burn is quickly 'relieved' through the oil
and warmth maintained deep into the treated part of
the body.

The use of essential oils includes additional thera-peutic effects. For example, lavender oil can be used for relaxation, or eucalyptus oil for stimulating breathing.

If the purpose is the diversion of metabolic processes from an infected area, or to increase consciousness and to have an incarnating effect, then no oil is applied.

Using mustard Mustard applications belong to the most effective and also to the most demanding of the external applica-tions. Knowing the indications and contra-indications gives confidence so that the compress may be applied without fear.

With this application it is especially important that the recipient has been well informed about the proc-ess and the expected burning effect. Such preparation makes it easier to cope with the experience of the first 'burning climax', and to tolerate the compress more comfortably for a longer period. Every therapy with mustard requires special care and guidance from the practitioner.

Duration The length of time for a mustard application must be individually decided. If the application is too short the required effect may not occur, and if too long a real dan-ger of a severe burn exists. Careful observation and good judgment of the situation is therefore very important.

The following points need to be observed. Depending on the recipient's condition or temperament, either encouragement towards holding out for longer or stop-ping earlier may be required. Sensitivity depends on the different skin types: people with blond or reddish hair often have a stronger skin reaction. Mustard tolerance is usually comparable to sun tolerance.

People who have sensitivity disorders, for example after a stroke, still experience an intense skin reaction and often burn much later. With such patients or with children, lift the compress after 5 to 10 minutes to see whether the skin has already become red, and decide whether to continue. In any case the compress should not remain on longer than 10 minutes the first time.

People who are not well incarnated or have a disturbed body sense, for example in the case of dissocia-
tive conditions, may not experience a burning sensation
or show a skin response. In this situation the application
should be stopped after 15 minutes. However, this does
not mean that the application has not had an effect.
Further observation regarding skin reaction and changes
experienced during following mustard applications can
greatly help the evaluation of an illness.

Mustard powder contains highly volatile etheric oil and **General point**
so should be kept in an airtight container away from
sunlight. It loses its efficacy with time, so old mustard
burns less intensely than fresh.

Mustard oils become active in contact with water.
They are quite resistant to heat, breaking down at about
70°C (160°F).

Chest and back compresses

Through the induced skin inflammation, metabolic
processes are diverted from infected lung areas onto
the skin. This release is experienced by many people as
opening up an 'inner realm' into which they are better
able to breathe.

After a mustard chest compress is completed, eucalyptus oil can be applied to continue the process. This
etheric oil prolongs the warmth effect, works against
infection and stimulates breathing.

Lung infections (pneumonia) **Indications**
Acute or chronic bronchitis
Spastic bronchitis; in this case a compress is usually given
    once or twice weekly

Skin damage, weeping or infected **Contra-indications**
Skin illnesses in the area of the compress
Redness not yet dissipated from a previous compress
Allergic reaction to mustard

Material For a back–compress about 100 g ($\frac{1}{2}$ cup) mustard powder
For a chest and back compress about 400 g (2 cups) mustard powder
Water 39–40°C (102–104°F)
Bowl
Mustard cloth known as envelope cloth, 2 to 3 times bigger than area to be treated
A thin layer of large tissue paper (about 100 × 50 cm, 40 × 20 in) or paper hand towels
Outer woollen cloth which can be generously wrapped around upper body
Inner cotton cloth which can be generously wrapped around upper body
Bed protection (to prevent leaking of mustard onto sheets)
For a chest compress, protection for the nipples even for men is important: tissue swab squares or gauze bandage
For a chest compress underarm protection may be provided with layers of tissue
Face–cloth
Diluted essential oil or neutral oil
Resting cloth with which the upper body may be generously covered

Preparation Just before it is required, open the mustard envelope cloth and put a piece of large tissue paper inside to spread the mustard on. This makes it easier to remove the mustard. Spread 2–3 mm ($\frac{1}{10}$ in) of mustard powder evenly over the tissue paper so as to cover the required part of the body. Then fold the tissue paper together to enclose all the mustard use medical tape to close the package. It is important that only one layer of material lies between the skin and the mustard. Take care not to leave parts of the cloth empty and unfolded, as this creates uncomfortable cold areas. The envelope is then carefully folded into a roll, making sure the mustard does not slip.

Procedure Lay the outer and inner cloths, together with the cloth protecting the bed, behind the sitting patient at shoulder level.

Cover the mustard compress in hot running water or put it into a shallow bowl so that it becomes evenly moist. Then without wringing, carefully press excess water out, the colour of the water should be yellow. The compress must be body temperature when applied.

A back compress is laid on the back and the patient lies down. The inner and outer cloths are wrapped around the chest and firmly tucked in.

A chest and back compress is rolled open to the width of the back and the patient lies down on it. Cover the nipples and underarms for protection before the compress is rolled from the sides over the chest. Cover with the inner and outer cloths and tuck in firmly.

Remain in the room with the patient during the compress, or make sure you are within calling distance.

Duration The duration can be between 5 and 20 minutes, depending on the recipient's experience of the compress, and is decided with the practitioner.

The first therapy with mustard is usually shorter as the burning often occurs surprisingly fast. If the patient is afraid or feels unsure, then it is better to stop the therapy. The subsequent therapy session can be longer if the person is happy with this and if the skin reaction from previous therapy is no longer visible.

For an intense effect a mustard chest compress may be given daily for three consecutive days.

Finishing off Remove the mustard compress. Carefully clean the skin with a warm face-cloth and dry using soft pressing movements. Afterwards a little oil can be spread on with a few slow movements and then wrap the patient in the rest cloth.

Clean the mustard cloth thoroughly using warm water, then wring and hang to dry. In time the compress cloth will become yellow and hard. A machine wash will be necessary after several uses.

Rest After every compress a rest is required of half an hour, this may be extended to an hour in some circumstances.

Onion *(Allium cepa)*

A fresh onion is cut in small pieces and wrapped in a thin, cotton cloth and applied for a number of hours.

Effect Onion contains strong sulfuric vitality and formative forces in balanced proportion. For this reason, the onion can release chronic blocked infectious processes and activate them, for example releasing mucus and pus secretions. Alternatively, if there is an active infectious process, the onion has a calming relaxing effect decreasing swelling and pain.

An onion cream could be used as a post therapy in mild cases or if there is a strong antipathy to onion.

Compresses for ear, chest or inflamed areas

Indications for ear compress Acute middle ear inflammation
It is important that the onion compress covers both the outer ear and the surrounding area of the temple to the hair-line. This compress often results in immediate pain relief and is very helpful with children for pain relief at night.

Indications for chest compress Bronchitis with extreme coughing and tacky mucus

Indications for inflamed areas Acute rheumatoid arthritis, inflamed synovial membranes
Painful upper leg
Tendinitis

Contra-indications Antipathy to onions or inability to cope with fumes
Skin infections or weeping wounds or cuts in the application area

Material One small onion or half a large onion is enough for an ear compress
Knife and chopping board
Thin cotton cloth, tape or thread
Cotton or unspun wool as padding

Small plastic bag and hot-waterbottle may be used if
  necessary
The outer cloth is either a scarf, hat, neck band or bandage such that the compress is held securely

Chop the onion into small pieces and spread about 1 **Procedure**
cm ($^1/_2$ in) thick on a thin cotton cloth of appropriate
size for the area being treated. Fold the sides inwards and
secure firmly so the contents are well contained. In the
case of a patient with fever or when treating a part of
the body sensitive to cold, the compress can be placed
in a plastic bag on a hot-waterbottle. Apply the onion
compress to the body, add a thick layer of wool as padding and secure firmly.

A number of hours, even overnight   **Duration**
  The compress develops an intense smell over this
time that some patients and those nearby find intolerable.

Cover the skin for several hours to protect from cold. **Finishing off**
  Wash the implements well, and dispose of the onion
compress.

Quarter to half an hour   **Rest time**

Potato *(Solanum tuberosum)*

Fresh boiled whole potatoes, with skin still attached are wrapped in a cloth and firmly pressed. This compress is applied as hot as is acceptable.

Effect Boiled potatoes maintain their heat over a long period. A potato application is deeply warming and subsequently has an analgesic and cramp-relieving effect.

Throat and chest compresses

Indications Inflamed throat with pain, when swallowing
Bronchitis with a cough that is deeply irritating and difficult to restrain; a continual coughing reflex

Contra-indications Skin infections, weeping wounds or cuts in the application area

Material Enough potatoes to cover the required area
Saucepan
Inner cloth, 2 to 3 times larger than the area being treated
Chopping board
Adhesive tape
An outer cloth

Preparation Boil unpeeled fresh potatoes for 45 minutes until soft. Drain the water and remove the lid to allow the potatoes to dry. Place the hot potatoes on the cotton inner cloth and pressed firmly with the wooden chopping board until about 1 cm ($^1/_2$ in) thick. Spread the potatoes to cover the area required. Fold the cloth and tape it down.

CAUTION Fresh cooked potatoes are very hot. Test the temperature of the compress on the forearm before application.

Roll the outer cloth from the outer edge inwards. Apply **Procedure**
the potato compress to the required area of the body,
wrap and secure the outer cloth firmly.

One hour or longer, as long as the compress remains **Duration**
warm and is experienced as pleasant and comfortable
for the recipient.

Cover the treated area with a thin cloth for several hours **Finishing off**
to protect from cold and draughts.
   Discard used potatoes. Wash the inner cloth and hang
out to dry with the outer cloths.

About half an hour, depending on the indications and **Rest time**
situation of the patient.

Quark

The quark is spread over a compress and left on until dry. Low fat quark is used from organic or Demeter sources, if available. Low fat quark is more suitable as it dries out quicker than high fat quark.

Essences can be added to the quark, such as arnica or meadowsweet essence, depending on the area of application and the required effect.

Effect Quark is prepared by separating soured milk into curds and whey. The firmer curds are the quark, while the fluid is the whey. This process of separating continues during the quark compress, with whey forming as the quark dries. This separation process creates a slow gentle drawing effect, with the watery whey relieving congestion and assisting removal of metabolic wastes from the body.

A quark application for an acute infection has a relieving, cooling, analgesic effect.

Compresses for inflamed and congested conditions

Indications Acne, abscesses, furuncles and venous infections (such as following an intravenous infusion)

Acute joint inflammation such as rheumatoid arthritis, hemarthrosis (blood effusion in a joint), inflammation of bursa membrane as in the knee and joint swellings following an operation

Oedematous swelling in the limbs resulting from a number of causes such as lymphatic congestion (arm or leg compress)

Congested lung conditions such as pleural effusion or lung infections (chest compress)

Ascites (abdominal compress)

CAUTION In chest conditions it is very important to observe the patient well during the quark treatment taking careful note of complaints of a sense of constraint, pressure or tightness in the chest and circulatory problems.

Allergy to lactic acid   **Contra-indications**

Usually a quark compress is given at body temperature, **Temperature** especially when applied on the trunk (back, chest and abdomen). For inflammations on the limbs or smaller areas it can be applied cooler.

   Never heat quark over 40°C *(104°F)* otherwise the protein in the quark coagulates and the whey separates and evaporates before the compress is applied.

250 g ($^1/_2$ lb) low fat quark for a 30 × 30 cm (12 × 12 **Materials** in) compress
Spatula or knife
Inner cloth: double layer material 2–3 cm (1 in) wider than the area being treated
Number of gauze compresses or a large piece of gauze fabric
Outer cloth that wraps around the area being treated generously
Elastic bandages as appropriate
Hot-waterbottles with plastic bags for protection (several hot-waterbottles may be required depending on the compress being prepared)
Bed protector
Face-cloth to clean the skin after the compress

Take the quark from the fridge some hours before **Preparation** application to allow it to settle at room temperature. Lay out the inner cloth and place a layer of gauze over it so that the quark is easily disposed of after the treatment. Spread the quark in a thick layer 3–5 mm ($^1/_4$ in) over the gauze cloth leaving the edge free of quark. Place a gauze compress over the quark to prevent too much quark being left on the skin.

   Warm the quark to body temperature for sensitive body parts by placing it on a hot-waterbottle that has been covered in a plastic bag to prevent staining.

Method Protect the bed and lay the outer cloth under the area being treated. Place the inner cloth (with quark) with the gauze side on the skin. Wrap the outer cloth firmly and secure well.

Duration This compress is left on for 1 to 4 hours, depending on the application area and the indications. It can be left on overnight. The quark should be dry and crumbly when removed.

Finishing off After removal of the compress, wash the body with warm water and dry.

Dispose of the quark compress. Rinse the inner cloth with cold water, then wash well with hot water. Wash the inner cloth thoroughly as any excess whey hardens and leaves a strong cheese aroma. Hang all cloths out to dry and air.

Clean hot-waterbottles well, removing any traces of quark.

Rest time Quarter to half an hour

Breast compress

Indications Inflamed breast tissue such as mastitis in breast-feeding women

As soon as the breast becomes hard, inflamed, painful or overly hot, apply this treatment. It is given after breast feeding and in acute situations applied after every feed. If after 24 hours there is no improvement, then consult a midwife or physician.

Usually the whole breast is treated. Occasionally, when there is a clearly defined inflammation a small compress is applied to the specific area.

The temperature of the compress for mastitis and breast infections is decided by the recipient. When a hot temperature is required then a mercurialis compress is used, while if a cooler temperature is required then the quark is applied at room temperature. In acute conditions, it is often beneficial to apply a hot mercurialis compress before the feed, and the quark compress after each feed.

The quark compress has a cooling, analgesic and anti- **Effect**
inflammatory effect.

The quark compress on the breast must be prepared **CAUTION**
hygienically to avoid aggravating fresh infections. Always
wash your hands before treatment and prepare a fresh
quark compress each time. Never reuse inner cloths.

    Never heat quark over 40°C (104°F) otherwise the
protein in the quark coagulates and the whey separates
and evaporates before the compress is applied.

Allergy to lactic acid **Contra-indications**

250 g ($^1/_2$ lb) low fat quark for a 30 × 30 cm (12 × 12 **Materials**
    in) compress
Spatula or knife
1 or 2 inner cloths: double layer material 2–3 cm (1 in)
    wider than the area being treated
Large piece of gauze fabric
Outer cloth that is 40 cm (16 in) wide and long enough
    to generously wrap around the chest
Elastic bandages as appropriate
1 or 2 hot-waterbottles with plastic bags for protection
Face-cloth to clean the skin after the compress

Take the quark from the fridge some hours before **Preparation**
application to allow it to settle at room temperature.
Cut the inner cloth in the middle to leave an opening, allowing the nipple to be free of quark. This is
important to prevent the skin becoming soft around
the nipple area.

    Lay out the inner cloth and place a layer of gauze
over it so that the quark is easily disposed of after the
treatment. Spread the quark in a thick layer 3–5 mm ($^1/_4$
in) over the gauze cloth leaving the edge free of quark.
Place a gauze compress over the quark to prevent too
much quark being left on the skin.

    Warm the compress a little by placing it on a hot-
waterbottle covered in a plastic bag to prevent staining.

Method Roll out the outer cloth behind the sitting recipient who then lies down. Depending on the requirement, treat either one or both breasts. Apply the inner cloth spread with quark, with the gauze side directly on the skin, avoiding touching the nipple area. The quark compress is at room temperature when applied, but if the recipient chooses it can be cooler. Wrap the outer cloth firmly around the recipient and secure well.

Duration This compress is left on for one or more hours. The quark should be dry and crumbly when removed.

Finishing off After removal of the compress, wash the body with warm water and dry.

Dispose of the quark compress. Rinse the inner cloth with cold water, then wash well with hot water. Wash the inner cloth thoroughly as any excess whey hardens and leaves a strong cheese aroma. Hang all cloths out to dry and air.

Clean hot-waterbottles well, removing any traces of quark.

Rest time Quarter to half an hour

Thuja leaf juice *(Thuja occidentalis)*

The thuja tree is an ancient conifer, with flat feathered leaves covered in green scales that contain many skin-irritating etheric oils, camphor and slimy gelatinous substances. Thuja contains strong, active life forces that can enliven a wound and encourage healing. It has a robust cleansing and antiseptic effect, even more than the calendula. This quality allows the effective release of foreign particles, as in the case of an infection.

Wound compress

Indications

Slow-healing, infected and putrid wounds lacking life vitality such as lower leg ulcer, bed sores, slow-healing perineum following episiotomy

Open, bleeding or infected nipples of breast-feeding women, ideally cleansing nipples with the juice before breast feeding

This compress can be used a number of times in the day, depending on what is required.

Contra-indications

Allergy to thuja

Materials for preparing fresh juice

4–8 fresh thuja leaf tips about 5 cm (2 in) long
Sharp knife and wooden chopping board
Mortar and pestle
Small bowl
Several large gauze dressings or pieces of muslin, as required
Glass jar or bottle that has been rinsed with boiled water and has a well sealed lid for the prepared juice

Materials for wound dressing

Combine dressings as required
Outer cloth or elastic bandage as appropriate
Disposable gloves as required

Preparation of juice

Wash the thuja leaf tips with warm water and place on a damp chopping board to retain the juices. Cut the leaf tips finely with a sharp knife. Then put them into the mortar and grind firmly with the pestle. Add a small quantity of fresh cold water, enough to cover the ground leaves. Leave for 15 to 20 minutes.

This slimy substance is further ground with the pestle to release more of the gelatinous material. Lay a dampened gauze dressing over the bowl and pour the contents of the mortar onto it. Squeeze the gauze well to release the thuja juices. Put the left-over slimy thuja substance into the mortar, add water, and grind with the pestle again, strain and re-squeeze through the gauze. Dip the remains of the slimy substance in the gauze into the water again and squeeze out well for a third time. Re-strain the juice through gauze into the storage bottle. Note the preparation date on the bottle and store in the fridge.

Freshly prepared thuja juice has a light green colour and a pleasantly fresh aroma. The prepared juice can be used for 2 to 3 days. After 2 days, the colour browns and it can still be used. Once the juice smells putrid, dispose of it.

Application Soak a gauze compress in the fresh juice and squeeze a little before placing over the wound. Additional compresses are used to cover and secure the wound. The compress is left on 10 to 30 minutes.

Normal awareness of wound hygiene is required. For infected wounds use disposable gloves.

Continue treatments as required.

Finishing off Dispose of the used gauze and thuja leftovers. Wash and dry the utensils.

Washing soda (Sodium carbonate)

The inner cloth is soaked in a washing soda solution and applied to the vertebrae at body temperature. This compress is normally applied on the thoracic and lumbar vertebrae.

Spinal compress

Washing soda activates and enlivens the nervous system **Effect**

Multiple sclerosis **Indication**

Skin damage, where there are weeping, infected skin **Contra-indication**
    lesions in the area of the compress application.

1 tbsp washing soda **Material**
300 ml (10 fl oz) water at 40°C (104°F)
Shallow bowl
Inner cloth 20 cm (8 in) wide and long enough to cover
    the affected area
Smaller outer cloth as wide as the back and 20 cm (8 in)
    longer than the inner cloth
Second outer cloth that is large enough to wrap gener-
    ously around the torso
Hot–waterbottle

For more details see *Liver, abdominal and kidney compresses* **Procedure**
on page 22.
    Fold the inner cloth in half, warm the outer cloth with a hot–waterbottle, and roll the second outer cloth from the outer edges towards the middle. The recipient rolls onto their side or sits upright. Unroll the second outer cloth behind their back and place on the bed with the smaller outer cloth on top.
    Pour hot water onto the washing soda and mix; soak the inner cloth in the solution, wring out well and lay on the smaller outer cloth. The recipient lies down on the compress and should experience the compress as

pleasantly warm. Draw the large outer cloth around the torso and wrap firmly.

If the recipient has a swayback place a small pillow under the compress, to ensure firm contact with the skin. If necessary position a knee roll under the knees for comfort. It is important that the covering blanket is firmly tucked around the body to provide a clear sense of boundary.

Duration 20 to 30 minutes

Rest Half hour

If during the rest there is a sense of restlessness in the legs or an unpleasant sensation is experienced in the spinal cord then discontinue this treatment.

Finishing off Remove the cloths, rinse the inner cloth and hang all cloth to air.

White cabbage *(Brassica oleracea)*

Fresh white cabbage leaves are applied for several hours. Savoy cabbage leaves can also be used.

White cabbage has a cooling relaxing effect on inflammatory processes and stimulates life forces. In the case of wounds with a lack of sensation, it can have an awakening effect that may result in pain. Hardened wounds can be softened, necrosis can be released and wound secretions activated. This can cause the wound to discharge heavily and stimulate wound cleansing, allowing healing.

Joint and wound compresses

Indications

Inflamed swollen joints, for example osteoarthritis and rheumatoid arthritis

Slow-healing necrotic wounds such as leg ulcers and bed sores

CAUTION

Cabbage leaves must only be applied over the open wound area because they weaken and damage healthy skin. Do not to apply cabbage leaves over the wound edges.

Materials

Cabbage head
Sharp knife
Chopping board with rolling pin
Hot-waterbottle and small plastic bag for protection, as necessary
Outer cloth and bandages
Neutral oil as required after a compress to joints

Method

Wash a number of juicy green cabbage leaves in warm water and dry. Remove the leaf spine and roll the leaves on the board with a rolling pin. Warm the leaves on a hot-waterbottle as needed, and apply to the required body part. Cover with a cloth or appropriate dressing, and secure with a bandage.

Duration The compress is applied for up to 12 hours, as long as it is experienced as comfortable by the recipient

Finishing off Wrap the cabbage head in a plastic bag and leave at room temperature rather than refrigerated. From experience it is more effective this way. Dispose of the used leaves.

In the case of very sensitive patients after the compress wash the skin with warm water and dry. Depending on the situation apply a neutral oil.

Rest time This is dependent on the indication and situation of the patient.

4

Lotions

A lotion is an alcoholic plant extract or an alcohol solution with mineral or animal substances. The lotion is usually diluted with water in a 1:40 or 1:50 solution.

The inner cloth is soaked in the diluted lotion either as a hot, wet treatment or less often a cold or warm treatment.

For measuring, note following:

   one teaspoon (tsp) is 5 ml

   one tablespoon (tbsp) is 15 ml

You may need a measuring cup or lotion bottle lid to measure the required amount of lotion.

Mix 6 ml of a 10% or 20% lotion with 300 ml (10 fl oz) water. This is sufficient to soak the cloth without superfluous fluid.

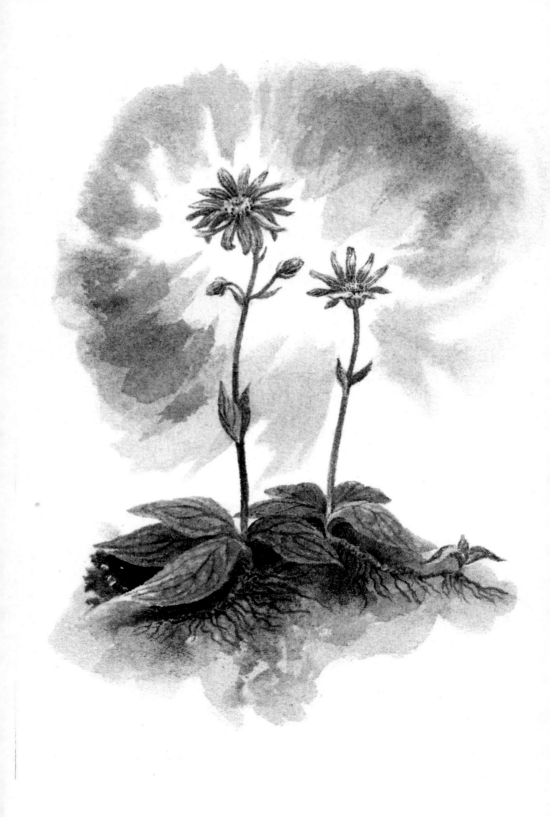

Arnica *(Arnica montana)*

Arnica is a plant of the mountains, growing solely on nutrient–poor, siliceous soils of upland meadows, as well as in moorlands or heaths.

It has a strong brown central root from which long, hard smaller roots enter the deeper layers of the earth. The root dies near its base, continually growing horizontally beneath the ground and forming nodes. From the nodes a rosette of leaves grows during spring and summer. The rosette consists of two or three opposite pairs of leaves. The leaves are ovoid, leathery and hard. In the following year a strong erect, unbranched stem grows. The stem may have two or more leaf pairs, and carries a single flower head. The stem has reddish hairs just beneath the primary flower.

Arnica flowers in summer, in Europe from early June to August. The flower heads rise above surrounding plants, proud and self–confident, strong, big and intensely yellow, reaching upwards. The irregular petals have an untidy appearance. Because of this rather lopsided and untidy flower head each arnica plant, despite the regularity of its developing shoots, has a very individual appearance. After flowering a 'dandelion like' seed head appears, rather wilder and less regular than that of the dandelion.

In the morning light the arnica flower looks towards the rising sun. This sensitivity to light together with the fine hairs over the whole plant indicates a strong silica process.

The stem and leaves are covered with a resinous furry texture that, when rubbed, release a warm, aromatic and pleasant smell on the hands. The flower has a warm, heavy, slightly bitter and spicy, rich aromatic smell. In arnica, right down to the roots, there are ample etheric oils, silicic acid, tannic acid, potash salts, resins and camphor–like substances.

Effect Arnica combines the silica formative forces seen in the stiff rigidity of the green stem with a dissipating warmth-tendency in the aroma of the untidy flower in a harmonious balance. Because of this, its effect can offer both structure and relief for cramps. It can bind the too strong forces of metabolism when there is an inflammation and, also dissolve the hardening forces of cramping. It combines a forming, binding with dissolving tendency.

Arnica represents a principle of forming that can re-enliven lost formative forces and return the right form again. The plant works through its strong vitality right into the nerve-sense system. It regulates irritations of the blood flow right up to the brain and harmonises the heart rhythm.

Contra-indications Allergy to arnica
Open tissues or weeping, inflamed skin

Caution Unfortunately arnica allergies are common and becoming more prevalent. Allergy can arise during a course of treatments or as a result of too strong a concentration of arnica lotion. The reaction begins as a small rash that increases and can develop into a swelling of the mucus membranes. If the treatment is stopped immediately symptoms will pass quickly.

Heart compress

Indications Irregular and too fast a pulse, arrhythmia
Heart failure or cardiac insufficiency
Cramp-like heart problems with feelings of fear and tension like angina attacks
Accompanying treatment after a heart attack
Unsettled heart caused by nervousness or weather sensitivity
Patients who feel their heart is too weak or beats uncomfortably hard or strong

The heart compress is applied very warm, 2–3°C, **Temperature**
(4–5°F) higher than body temperature. In cases of
cramp-like or angina heart problems use as hot as possible.

It is important with a heart compress that the patient **Caution**
experiences its duration and temperature as pleasantly
and as beneficially as possible.

6 ml 20% arnica lotion **Material**
200 ml (7 fl oz) water at 40–43°C (104–110°F) or hotter
Shallow bowl
Inner cloth
Outer cloth 30 × 40 cm (12 × 16 in)

Fold the inner cloth to 20 × 30 cm (8 × 12), dip it in **Procedure**
the bowl of lotion and water. Wring it well, and quickly
place it over the heart area. Cover with the outer cloth.

Half to one hour **Duration**
   If patient falls asleep leave the compress *in situ*. Take
the hot compress off as soon as it cools, and repeat if
required.

Remove all cloths, rinse the inner cloth, dry and air. **Finishing off**

Quarter to half an hour **Rest time**

Forehead compress

Headaches, for instance nervousness or sensitivity to **Indications**
   weather
Knock to head or concussion

6 ml 20% arnica lotion **Material**
200 ml (7 fl oz) water (cool to warm)
Shallow bowl
Inner cloth
Outer cloth 15 cm (6 in) wide, long enough to gener-
   ously go around the head

Safety pins
Protective covering for pillow

Temperature The temperature can be cool or warm depending on the patient's preference or medical prescription.

Procedure Fold inner cloth to 10 cm (4 in) width. It needs to be long enough to reach across forehead from ear to ear, covering the temples. Put protective covering on the pillow. Prepare the lotion and water in the bowl. Dip the inner cloth in bowl, wring well and place on forehead. Quickly wrap the outer cloth around the head and secure with safety pins.

Duration Quarter to three quarters of an hour.

Finishing off Remove cloths and rinse. Hang up all cloths to dry and air.

Rest time Quarter to half an hour

Wrist or ankle cloth

Indications Collapse or tendency to collapse. In this case the cloth is put on as hot as possible and removed as soon as it starts to cool. It will help the patient to be more wakeful. Repeat as needed.
Crisis with hypertonia: these patients often have a red, blocked-up sensation in the head
Sudden tachycardia

Material 6 ml 20% arnica lotion
200 ml (7 fl oz) water
Shallow bowl
2 inner cloths
2 outer cloths, each 15–20 cm (6–8 in) wide, so the wrist is well covered

Temperature Depending on the patient's need in the last two cases compresses are put on either 1–2°C (2–4°F) higher or lower than the body temperature, comfortably warm.

Roll the inner cloth into a width of 10 cm (4 in) and **Procedure**
also roll in the outer cloth from the sides. Add the lotion
to the water in the bowl. Soak the inner cloth, wring
it out and place around the wrists or ankles quickly.
Completely cover with the outer cloth and secure with
safety pins. This compress encompasses the pulse points
of either wrists or ankles.

Quarter to three quarters of an hour.   **Duration**

Remove cloths and rinse. Hang up all cloths to dry and **Finishing off**
air.

Quarter to half an hour   **Rest time**

Arm wrap

Paralysis, stroke or loss of awareness of limbs   **Indications**
This wrap is done at a pleasantly warm temperature.

6 ml arnica 20 % lotion   **Material**
200 ml (7 fl oz) water
Shallow bowl
Inner and outer cloth
Safety pins
Large towel to protect bed
Covered hot-waterbottles, about 40°C (104°F)

Roll in inner and outer cloths. Put protective towel **Procedure**
under the arm. Mix lotion in water, dip inner cloth and
wring well. Wrap the whole arm from the fingertips
to the shoulder. Wrap the outer cloth around quickly
and smoothly, so inner cloth maintains its temperature.
Check there are no wrinkles or openings at the ends to
avoid air cooling the cloth.

   Depending on patient's feeling, place hot-waterbottles as necessary.

Quarter to three quarters of an hour.   **Duration**

Finishing off Remove cloths and rinse. Hang up all cloths to dry and air.

Rest time Quarter to half an hour

Wraps & compresses for bruises & traumas

Indications Bruised or strained joint
Bruised skin (not open wound)
Hematoma, post operative swellings
Arnica cream or arnica gel can be used alternatively with the wrap or compress.

Caution Arnica essence must not be used on open wounds.

Temperature Acute injuries, if the wound is hot or swollen, put the compress on cool. This causes a drawing in of the blood vessels and reduces the swelling. If possible elevate the injured area.
    On an older wound use a hot to warm compress, depending on the patient's need.

Material 6 ml 20% arnica lotion
200 ml (7 fl oz) water
Shallow bowl
Inner and outer cloths

Procedure Prepare the inner cloth to appropriate size. Add lotion to water in bowl. Dip inner cloth, wring well and apply. Put on outer cloth and secure with safety pin.

Duration Quarter to three quarters of an hour.

Finishing off Remove cloths and rinse. Hang up all cloths to dry and air.

Rest time Quarter to half an hour

Head cap

Apoplexy, stroke **Indications**

6 ml 20% arnica lotion **Material**
200 ml (7 fl oz) water
Inner cloth, big enough to wrap several times around
    the head including hair and ears
Outer cloth of similar size
Safety pins
Towel to protect the bed

The wrap should be pleasantly warm for the patient **Temperature**

Put the protection on pillow. Mix lotion in bowl, dip **Procedure**
the inner cloth, soak and squeeze well. Wrap quickly
round head, add the outer cloth, wrap quickly and
secure firmly.

Quarter to three quarters of an hour. **Duration**

Remove cloths and rinse. Hang up all cloths to dry and **Finishing off**
air.

Quarter to half an hour **Rest time**

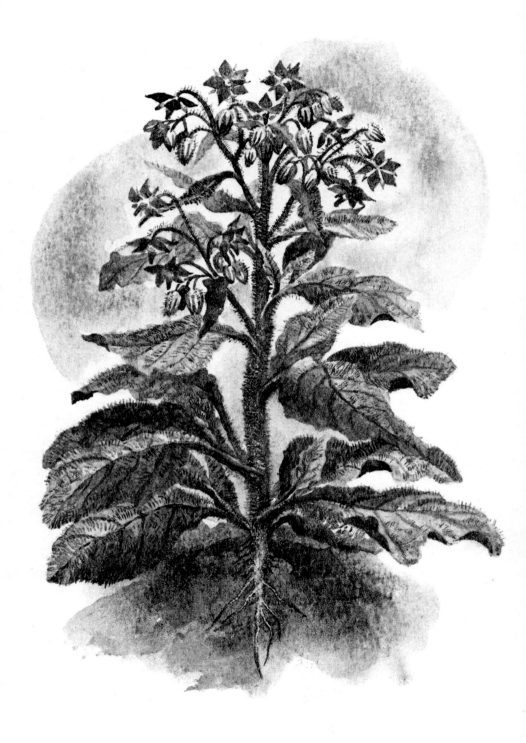

Borage *(Borago officinalis)*

Borage is grown in many home gardens, originally coming from the Mediterranean. It is found in sunny, light filled areas alongside dry ditches and embankments. Borage has a light–coloured, hard tap root that rapidly develops a number of large, simply formed green/grey oval leaves prior to the stem development. The stem is succulent, sappy, soft and quickly branches upwards to the sun. In rich, moist soil the plant spreads its leaves abundantly. The plant is covered in fine, prickly, silver hairs.

At the top of the stems, a number of rich flower buds hang tightly together like little protected bundles. One after another the buds open and flower for a short period of time. The flowers are a soft pink changing to an intense blue colour before wilting. Each flower has five petals, forming a clear geometric star. Between the petals the fine sepals can be seen radiating outwards. In the middle of the flower are dark, almost black stamens protruding like prickles.

Borage blooms almost continuously throughout the three months of summer, new blossoms always appearing on fresh side–shoots. Like most of the Boraginaceae family it attracts many bees through its plentiful nectar production.

Although the stem and leaves have a covering of rough hair–like prickles they are still quite succulent. They taste fresh, cool and cucumber–like; the smell is sweet and refreshing.

The borage plant remains green and succulent despite its sunny, dry position in the garden and it never seems to dry out. Rather than a fiery flowering quality, borage has its vitality in the leaf region, while the flowers rest on quiet, cool stalks. The flowers are like soft, sky-blue stars peacefully resting above the rich leafy undergrowth. This plant radiates a peaceful almost melancholic mood. One of its names is the 'peaceful herb' and it is used for heavy moods, anxiety and nervousness. In borage there is no etheric oil, rather it has mucilage, tannins, saponins, silicic acid, and potash.

Effect In the case of an infection, when the metabolic processes are too active and fiery, borage has a cooling and calming effect; it is able to bring back forming qualities that relieves congestion and inflammation. Borage returns the natural balance and flow of fluids in the tissues.

Leg compress

Indications Venous inflammation (thrombophlebitis)
Venous clot (thrombosis)

Contra-indications Allergy to borage
Open tissues or weeping, inflamed skin

Temperature Apply warm, if there is a lack of circulation, or the legs are cold and oedematous. Apply cool, if there is inflammation or the legs are hot. Adapt the temperature to the patient's requirements and comfort. If uncertain consult a physician.

Material 6 ml borage 20% lotion
300 ml (10 fl oz) warm or cool water
Shallow bowl
Inner cotton bandage, compress or sock large enough to cover the required area; if the compress is up to the hip 2 or 3 may be required (see *Required Materials,* page 19)
Outer binder, bandage or sock (see *Required Materials*)
Bed protection as appropriate
Hot-waterbottles for hot compresses at approximately 40°C (104°F)

Preparation Prepare all inner cloths, roll or fold as appropriate. Similarly prepare the outer cloths. Protect the bed with plastic as appropriate.

Procedure Always include the foot in the compress that extends up the leg either to the knee or to the hip, ensuring the toes are not wrapped too tightly and have adequate space to move.

Depending on the situation or patient's condition, a second person may be needed to hold the leg while the compress is applied.

Prepare the lotion in the bowl at the required temperature. Soak the inner compress in the solution, squeeze well and apply from the toes to the knee or hip.

If the compress is warm, ensure it does not cool too quickly, wrapping the outer cloth quickly and firmly with overlaps of 2–4 cm (1–1½ in). The outer cloth can even be pre-warmed.

For a quick, effective leg wrapping using the minimum amount of cloth the following wrapping technique is shown for the outer cloth (see also diagram). Open the beginning of the outer cloth about 20 cm (8 in) and placed under the sole of the foot.

Fold the top corner of the cloth over the toes and edge of the foot. Then wrap the cloth around the leg avoiding any open folds that will trap cold air.

If the compress goes to the hip, soak the second inner cloth and follow on from the first cloth. Again wrap the outer cloth firmly around, following the inner cloth to the hip. If necessary, use a third cloth.

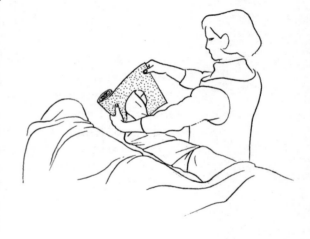

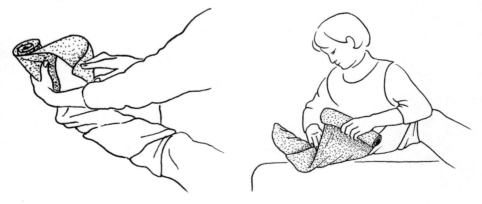

Prepare a fresh mixture of lotion in water for the second leg, and use the same procedure as for the first.

Use hot-waterbottles for the feet or beside the legs if required.

Duration Half to two hours, as required.

Finishing off Remove all cloths. Rinse the inner cloths with warm water and hang to dry. Hang the outer cloths to dry or air as required.

Rest Quarter to half an hour

Leg compress with borage mix

This leg compress is applied in the same manner as the borage leg compress. The mix comprises borage lotion with burdock root *(Radix bardanae* or *Radix lappa)* 10% and blackthorn or sloe *(Prunus spinosa)* 10%. This has an enlivening and activating effect on congested legs for a variety of causes. A lemon can also be added to this mixture.

Prepare lemon water so that the etheric oils are used as they have a healing effect (see *Preparation of lemon water,* page 69). If organic or unsprayed lemon is unavailable then use the juice of half a lemon.

Copper sulfate (cuprum sulfuricum)

Copper has a warming effect and regenerates the kidneys. The sulfur enhances this effect.

Kidney compress

Constitutional kidney problems **Indications**
High blood pressure caused by kidneys
Damaged kidneys from diabetes mellitus
The compress is done early in the morning because then it can support the kidney which becomes more active on waking.

Allergy or intolerance to copper sulfate **Contra-indications**
Commencement of menstruation, as it may be uncomfortable for some patients
Open wounds or skin irritations where the compress is to be applied to the kidneys

Wear gloves when using copper sulfate because it stains **Caution** the fingers blue.

6 ml copper sulfate 20% lotion **Material**
300 ml (10 fl oz) water at 40–42°C (104–108°F)
Shallow bowl
Inner cloth 20 × 30 cm (8 × 12 in)
Wool and cotton outer binders
Hot-waterbottles at about 40°C (104°F) with covers (for the feet and binders)
Plastic or rubber gloves

For a full description see *Liver, abdominal and kidney com-* **Procedure**
presses on page 22.
   Fold the inner cloth together. Roll the outer cloths from the outer edge towards the middle and pre-warm with a hot-waterbottle. Prepare the lotion mixture in the bowl.
   Roll out the outer cloths behind the sitting patient. Soak the inner cloth in the lotion mixture, wring out

well, and lay on the outer cloth. Hold all the cloths over the kidney area; the compress should be felt as pleasantly warm by the patient, 2–3°C (4–5°F) higher than body temperature.

The patient lies down and the outer cloths are wrapped around firmly. Place a hot-waterbottle on each side of the kidneys. Patients who have a hollow back may need a small pillow to ensure the inner cloth touches the kidney area.

Duration Half to three-quarters of an hour

Finishing off Remove the inner cloth, wash in warm water, and hang to dry.

Rest Quarter to half an hour

Formica *(Formica rufa)*

Red or wood ants are very important for the health, energy and life vitality of forests, especially because the formic acid they produce enlivens dead matter so it can be reabsorbed into the life processes of the forest. In the human organism formic acid is able to release sclerotic hardenings and deposits in the metabolic system allowing them to be reabsorbed in a healthy, structured manner.

Heart compress

Follow-up treatment after heart attack

Chronic sclerotic hardening processes in heart such as
    coronary heart disease

The heart compress can be applied at any time of the day, as required.

Indications

Allergy or inability to cope with formica

Weeping, infected skin lesions in the area of the compress application.

Contra-indications

8 ml formica 1% lotion

200 ml (7 fl oz) water at 40°C (104°F)

Small bowl

Inner cloth folded 20 × 30 cm (8 × 12 in)

Outer cloth, 30 × 40 cm (12 × 16 in) made of light, warm material

Material

It is especially important with the heart compress that it is experienced by the patient as comfortable and beneficial in respect of temperature and length of time.

    Mix the water and lotion in the bowl. Soak the inner cloth in the solution, wring out well and apply over the heart. It is important that the inner cloth is very warm, at least 2–3°C (4–5°F) warmer than the body temperature. Apply the outer cloth over the inner cloth.

Procedure

Liver of sulfur *(Hepar sulfuris)*

Liver of sulfur or hepar sulfuris is a mixture of various potassium sulfide salts, some of volcanic origin.

Sulfur has strong warmth within it that is released when it burns. The Latin *sol ferro,* meaning sun-carrier or carrier of the sun, is perhaps related to the word *sulfur,* and characterises the nature of this element. It carries pent-up volcanic heat, and is able to activate and bring warmth back to blocked metabolic processes. The warmth has the ability to revitalise the digestive system's natural rhythms. Potassium has an enlivening and invigorating effect on the etheric body.

Liver compress

Indications Hardening tendencies in the liver, for instance liver cirrhosis

Activation of metabolic processes in the digestion

Chronic long standing depressive conditions

This compress is applied as soon as possible after the midday meal in order to support the healthy metabolic activity of the liver.

Contra-indications First day of menstruation (a hot treatment to the abdomen can result in heavy bleeding)

Sulfur intolerance or even antipathy to the aroma

Skin infections, suppurations and irritations in the liver region

CAUTION Potassium sulfide solution smells like rotten eggs. Use disposable gloves to wring out the inner cloth.

To avoid having to place the inner cloth on a hot-waterbottle, wring it out close to the patient, to maintain heat.

Material 6 ml Liver of sulfur 30% lotion

300 ml (10 fl oz) hot water at about 75°C (170°F)

Shallow bowl

Inner cloth, 20 × 30 cm (8 × 12 in)

Wringing-cloth
Disposable rubber or latex gloves
Outer cloths large enough to wrap generously around
   the abdomen
Hot-waterbottle covered

See description of *Liver, abdominal and kidney compresses* **Procedure**
on page 22.

    The inner cloth is folded and rolled in the wringing-cloth. Roll the outer cloth from the sides into the centre, and place a hot-waterbottle in the middle to pre-warm it. Lay the outer cloth behind the back of the sitting recipient, who then lies back on the bed.

    Mix the lotion and water in the bowl, and soak the inner cloth inside the wringing-cloth. Wring them out well, quickly remove the inner cloth from the wringing-cloth, and placed as hot as possible on the liver region. Immediately wrap the outer cloth firmly around the abdomen to hold the inner cloth in position. Place a hot-waterbottle over the compress.

Half to three-quarters of an hour   **Duration**

Remove the cloths, rinse the bowl and the inner cloth, **Finishing off**
and hang all the cloths to dry.

Quarter to half an hour   **Rest**

Meadowsweet *(Filipendula ulmaria)*

This plant has many small, sweet smelling flowers, with white petals that give off a sweet aroma. It gives freshly mown hay its characteristic sweet smell. Meadowsweet contains many different etheric oils that extend right to the roots and carry different types of salicylic acid. Aspirin is the generic medical name for the chemical acetylsalicylic acid, a derivative of salicylic acid. *Acetyl* and *spirea* inspired the name aspirin.

Meadowsweet has an analgesic, anti–inflammatory, antipyretic effect and reduces swelling.

Joint compress

Indications Inflamed and painful joints for example joint inflammation such as osteoarthritis or rheumatoid arthritis.

Temperature Apply this compress cooler on hot and inflamed joints. For cold joints it may be applied warmer. However the temperature is adapted according to what is experienced by the patient as comfortable and pleasant.

Contra-indications Allergies to meadowsweet
Weeping wounds in the area to be treated

Material 6 ml meadowsweet 20% lotion
200 ml (7 fl oz) water, either hot or body temperature as required
Inner cloth
Outer cloth, which is large enough to be generously wrapped around the joint

Procedure Roll up the inner and outer cloths separately. Mix the lotion in the bowl. Soak the inner cloth in the diluted lotion, wring out well, and then apply around the joint. If treating the wrist or ankle the whole hand or foot is included in the compress. As soon as the compress is applied, quickly wrap the outer cloth and secure firmly.

Half an hour to an hour **Duration**

Remove the inner cloth. Cover the joint with a thin **Finishing off**
cloth for a while to protect from cold and draughts.
Wash the inner cloth with warm water, wring and
hang to dry. Air the outer cloth.

Quarter to half an hour **Rest**

Mercurialis *(Mercurialis perennis)*

Mercurialis perennis (sometimes known as dog's mercury) has a rhythmical, form, with dark-green coloured leaves and small inconspicuous green flowers. It is a vigorous, tenacious plant, with a widely branching perennial rhizome that holds a blue-coloured substance. This plant rightly carries the name of the healing god Mercury; with its strong wound healing, cleansing and anti-inflammatory properties.

Breast-tissue compress

This compress, when applied hot has a strong activating effect on the flow of breast milk. Hardened, restricted and inflamed areas in the breast tissue are relieved by this compress.

Indications Milk congestion
Breast tissue inflammation or mastitis
Use immediately when breast tissue hardens, is painful or develops inflamed areas. Ideally, apply directly prior to breast feeding. It can be used a number of times each day, if necessary prior to each feed. If there is no improvement within 24 hours consult a midwife or physician. Usually, both breasts are treated at the same time.

The decision on whether to use a hot, mercurialis or cool, quark compress depends on the recipient's preference; on whether the heat stimulates the milk flow or the cool anti-inflammatory quark is the most effective. The compresses could be used alternately, with the hot mercurialis before feeds and the cool quark following the feed.

Caution With this compress it is essential to follow proper hygiene procedures, to avoid further infection. Wash the bowl with boiling water prior to use, wash hands well, and change the inner and wringing towel every 24 hours.

6 ml mercurialis 20% lotion   **Material**
300 ml (10 fl oz) boiling water
Shallow bowl
2 inner cloths or a specially prepared breast cloths
2 wringing–cloths
Outer binder, 40 cm (16 in) wide and long enough to
    wrap around the recipient's chest
2 covered hot–waterbottles

See description of *Liver, abdominal and kidney compresses* **Preparation**
on page 22.
    Fold each inner cloth a number of times so it is thick
and large enough to cover the breast, then roll each and
place one in each wringing–cloth. Roll the outer binder
in from the sides, put a hot–waterbottle in the middle,
and placed on the bed.

Place the outer binder behind the back of the sitting **Procedure**
recipient, who then lies down on it. Prepare the lotion
in the bowl and place both combined cloths in the
solution. Wring out one compress firmly, and place
the inner cloth on the breast. Make sure the compress
does not touch the nipple as it should not be softened.
Quickly cover with the outer binder.
    Treat the other breast in the same way. Secure the
outer cloth firmly. Place a hot–waterbottle on each side
of the chest.

Half an hour to an hour   **Duration**

Remove both cloths. Wash the compress cloth with **Finishing off**
warm water, wring and hang to dry. Air the outer cloth.

No rest time is required as breast feeding normally fol– **Rest**
lows this treatment.

Wound compress

A gauze dressing soaked in the mercurialis solution is applied to the wound area. Normal hygienic practices must be maintained depending on the nature of the wound and situation.

Other lotions such as *Calendula officinale* and *Aristolochia clematitis* may be used.

Indications Wounds of varied types, like lower leg ulcers, pressure sores, open wounds on the chest such as in breast cancer

Contra-indications Allergy to the lotion

Material Mercurialis 20% lotion in normal saline 1:10 solution
Bowl and syringe to mix solution
Several gauze dressings
Outer binder or bandage with fastener
Bed protection

Procedure Mix the lotion as required; usually 1:10 solution is used. Never prepare more than is required for one day as the alcohol in this mix affects plastic, changing its quality and cleanliness.

Soak the compress in the solution, lightly squeeze and lay on the wound slightly moist. Cover with several gauze pads and bandage securely.

Duration Half to three quarters of an hour

Finishing off Remove the gauze dressings and dispose of them. Dress the wound as required.

Orthoclase (potassium feldspar)

Orthoclase (potassium or alkali feldspar) is a common constituent of granite, and can also be found as a crystal.

Heart compress

Silicon is receptive to cosmic forming energy. This quality is used for infections when there is a loss of formative energy and cellular structure. Orthoclase also gives enlivening and elasticity qualities.

Acute and chronic heart muscle infection (myocarditis) **Indications**
Patients experiencing restless heart symptoms
'Aging heart,' with a lack of vitality
This compress can be given at any time of day, and may be applied twice daily.

These compresses have the greatest effect when applied **Temperature**
cold. However, if experienced as uncomfortable they can be applied lukewarm to avoid a shock or trauma.

Allergy or sensitivity to orthoclase **Contra-indications**
Skin infections or weeping wounds in the heart area

20 ml orthoclase 0.1% lotion **Material**
200 ml (7 fl oz) water at 25–35°C (75–95°F)
Inner cloth
Outer cloth, about 30 × 40 cm (12 × 16 in), mad of a
   light, warm material
Bowl

For a heart compress it is especially important that the **Procedure**
patient's experience is pleasant and comfortable.
   Fold the inner cloth to about 20 × 30 cm (8 × 12 in). Mix the lotion in the bowl, soak the inner cloth and wring out well. Place it over the heart. Lay the outer cloth on top and cover with bedding.

Duration Half an hour to an hour

Finishing off Remove the cloths, wash the inner cloth, and hang to
dry with the outer cloth.

Rest Quarter to half an hour

Oxalis *(Oxalis acetosella)*

Common wood sorrel or shamrock, *Oxalis acetosella,* is a forest plant that grows in moist, cool shady ground, covering rotting pieces of trees, leaves and stones with its clover-like leaves. The roots are delicate and fibrous, spreading superficially over the ground barely connected with the earth. The stalks are 5 to 10 cm (2–4 in) long and have three heart-shaped leaves. The stalks at the base are a tender rose colour and the root is dark red.

Wood sorrel begins growth early spring and continues to grow to late autumn. The young leaves initially have a shiny, luminous spring green colour that later turns to a dark green often remaining through the winter, for they are quite tough. The leaves have a rare and unusual trait. When touched, or in strong wind, rain or bright sunlight the leaves of the plant fold down towards the stem, resulting in a thin, spindly appearance where there had been a rich, green covering.

In spring tender whitish flowers with fine violet veins appear out of the green leafy cover. The flowers contain a lot of nectar so bees and bugs like to visit them. Few seeds are formed from these early flowers. In summer there is a second flowering when smaller self-pollinating flowers develop with many seeds.

Wood sorrel has a very delicate and tender appearance. The horizontal spread leaves seem to be weightless and the stem so thin and delicate it is almost invisible; threefold leaves look like green drops floating on the surface of water. The plant has a sour fresh taste; it should not be eaten in great quantities as it contains oxalic acid.

Effect Wood sorrel possesses a strong vegetative force. The element of flowering, colour and movement is delicately woven into the plant life without overpowering the whole vegetative life. After flowering and seeding, the oxalis continues to grow. It is a most harmonious plant. Oxalis acts rather like ants with their formic acid, as it transforms decaying material into humus, returning it to

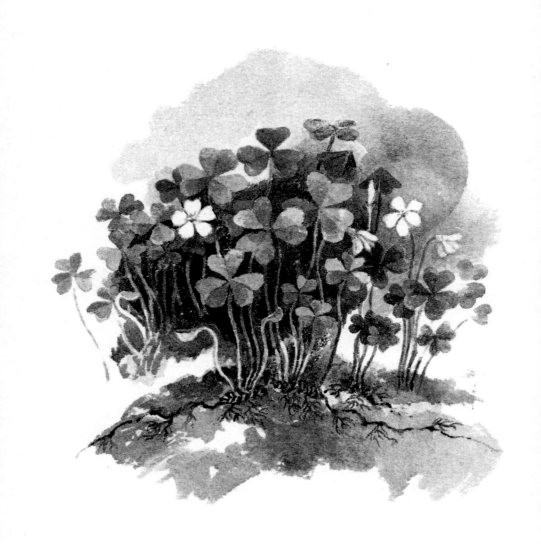

the life cycle. It transforms what is dead, returning it to an active life process.

Oxalis strengthens the life forces. (Beekeepers sometimes use formic or oxalic acid to strengthen the bees' immune system, protecting them from the varroa mite.) If someone has been torn apart by shock oxalis helps the soul spiritual being reintegrate and connect with the physical. It also supports the building up (anabolic) activity of the metabolic digestive processes so that food taken in can be assimilated into the organism.

Abdominal compress

After a shock or traumatic experience
Nervous disturbances in the digestive system
This compress is normally given in the evening before sleep

Indications for upper abdominal compress

Weakened exhausted patients
Poorly nourished patients, anorexia
Digestive difficulties resulting in weakened metabolism
Unspecific abdominal pains
Menstrual discomfort so long as it is comfortable having
   a compress on the abdomen
 This compress is normally given after the main midday meal

Indications for lower abdominal compress

Allergy to oxalis
Bruised abdomen or open, weeping, inflamed skin conditions in area being treated

Contra-indications

6 ml oxalis 20% lotion
300 ml (10 fl oz) water at 38–40°C (100–104°F)
Bowl
Inner compress cloth
Outer woollen and inner cotton cloth
Safety pins
Hot-waterbottle (slightly warmer than body temperature, about 38°C, 100°F)

Material

Procedure See description of *Liver, abdominal and kidney compresses* on page 22.

Fold the inner cloth to 20 × 30 cm (8 × 12 in) and roll the outer cloths towards the middle, pre-warming them with a hot-waterbottle.

Open the outer cloth behind the sitting patient who then lies on it. Mix the lotion. Soak the inner cloth, wring out and placed on the stomach. It should be at body temperature and be experienced as warm and pleasant. Wrap the outer cloth firmly and secure with a safety pin. Put a hot-waterbottle on the abdomen as desired. Support the knees with a roll if required.

Duration Half to three quarters of an hour

Finishing off Remove the inner cloth and rinse.

Rest Quarter to half an hour

5

Oil Cloths

An oil cloth is a cloth coated in oil that is warmed and applied for a number of hours, with padding to maintain warmth.

This form of oil application is used when a soft warm- **Indication**
ing effect is required. It is given over a number of hours and is ideal for painful or touch-sensitive areas when a rhythmic einreibung* is not suitable. An oil cloth provides mild warmth and is one of the comfortable pleasant and gentle therapies. It can easily be used in the home setting.

A variety of oils are used containing neutral, fatty based **Effect**
oil, such as olive, almond or peanut oil, mixed with an etheric oil or a plant extract. The fatty oils are derived from plants that have absorbed sunlight and warmth and thus have the quality of maintaining warmth over extended periods. Because of this quality, oil cloths pro-vide a warmth shield that re-enlivens and heals chronic cold or hardening processes. In addition, there is the specific healing effect from the etheric oil or plant sub-stance in the oil.

Oil cloths are usually given at night. Depending on the **Time of treatment**
condition they may be given at other times.

Allergy to the plant substance or oil base used   **Contra-indications**
Weeping, infected skin lesions in the area of the oil
    cloth application

* Rhythmic einreibung is a form of massage used in anthroposophical nursing. Its techniques were developed by the physicians Margarethe Hauschka, based on suggestions by Ita Wegman. See Fingado's compan-ion book, *Rhythmic Einreibung*.

Material Prescribed oil
Inner cloth: double layered material of the required size
Small plastic bag
Outer cloth that can be securely wrapped (may be firm-
fitting clothing)
Padding that 2–3 cm (1 in) larger than the oil cloth
Hot-waterbottle (warm or hot depending on the situation)

Padding Padding is used over the oil cloth to maintain the
warmth as long as possible. The padding is made out
of material that is not absorbent, is warming and well
ventilated. Cotton wool or a clean sheep's fleece that
still has lanolin present is often used. Wrap the padding
in muslin or a thin cotton cloth and secure as necessary.

Preparation Soak the inner cloth fully and evenly in the prescribed
oil. The first time the cloth is used the oil is only slowly
absorbed into the dry material. Place the cloth in a
plastic bag and warm on a hot-waterbottle, which helps
disperse the oil evenly into the oil cloth. Add oil until
the cloth is saturated.

Following each treatment, add a small amount of oil
to the cloth. The cloth always needs to be saturated and
have the aroma of the etheric oil that is being applied.

Immediately before a treatment, warm the oil cloth
in a plastic bag and along with the padding and outer
cloth on a hot-waterbottle, leaving it until it is 2–3°C
(3–5°F) above body temperature. The oil cloth should
feel pleasantly warm to the recipient.

CAUTION The oil cloth must not be warmed too much because
the oil quickly becomes rancid and the etheric oils are
damaged.

Procedure Remove the oil cloth from the plastic bag. Place it with
the padding on the area to be treated. Wrap the outer
cloth around and secure firmly to keep the oil cloth in
place. Generally, a hot-waterbottle is not required.

The oil cloth can be applied for a number of hours,
but the recipient must not perspire during this treatment.

Remove the oil cloth and keep the treated area warm **Finishing off**
with a warm cloth or clothing to protect against cooling
and draughts.

Store the oil cloth in a sealable plastic bag because oil
quickly becomes rancid when open to the air, and the
etheric oils evaporate.

An oil cloth can be used a number of times unless it
has an unpleasant aroma or seems to be aged. Depending
on the part of the body being treated or the skin type
the oil cloth may be used daily for 2 to 3 weeks.

Quarter to half an hour   **Rest time**

Aconite in olive oil (Oleum Aconitum napellus *3% or 5%)*

Aconite (monkshood) oil is often combined with other
oils such as Wala aconite nerve oil that has added camphor and lavender.

This oil has a relaxing effect on agitated nerves.   **Effect**

Pain from agitated nerves such as caused by neuralgia   **Indications**
Pain in all areas of the body, where there is tension and
    joint discomfort

Dependent on situation or condition.   **Size of cloth**

Caraway in olive oil (Oleum Carum carvi *10%)*

Relief of cramp and bloating   **Effect**

Bloating and flatulence   **Indications**
Cramping in the stomach–intestinal tract

20 × 30 cm (8 × 12 in)   **Size of cloth**

Camomile in olive oil (Oleum Chamomilla 10%)

Effect Deeply warming and cramp relieving

Indications Painful, cramping in stomach-intestinal area
Nervous restlessness at night
Cramping premenstrual discomfort

Size of cloth 20 × 30 cm (8 × 12 in)

Eucalyptus in olive oil (Oleum Eucaplypti 3%)

Effect Eucalyptus oil has a deeply warming effect that enables it to relax and relieve cramping of the bladder muscles. This oil also has an anti-inflammatory effect.

Indications Acute and chronic bladder infections (cystitis)
Nervous irritable bladder that leads to frequent urination at night

Method Depending on the situation, a warm hot-waterbottle can be placed on top of the oil cloth to provide additional relief of pain and cramping.
    Weleda eucalyptus 5% dispersion oil is a good substitute.

Size of cloth 15 × 20 cm (6 × 8 in)

Lavender in olive oil (Oleum Lavendulae 3%)

Lavender oil provides mild warmth that relaxes over **Effect**
stimulated nerves. It has a relaxing and harmonising
effect.

Bronchitis with an irritating dry cough   **Indications**
Convalescence from lung infections such as pneumonia,
    especially suitable for children
Painful ribs from frequent coughing
Spastic bronchitis

The oil cloth is placed on the appropriate area: ribs, **Procedure**
bronchial, chest or torso.
    Weleda lavender 10% dispersion bath oil is a good
substitute.

Dependent on situation and whether the cloth is to **Size of cloth**
encompass the whole chest or torso or treat a specific
part.

Solum uliginosum oil

This oil contains bog extract *(Solum uliginosum)*, chest-
nut *(Aesculus)*, equisetum or horsetail *(Equisetum arvense)*
and lavender oil and is manufactured by Wala.

Solum uliginosum oil conveys comfortable and encom- **Effect**
passing warmth, with a relaxing and relieving effect. It is
very effective for releasing and soothing tension in the
back, neck and shoulders.

Painful muscle tension, low back pain (lumbago) and **Indications**
    chronic painful conditions
Nerve pain (neuralgia) such as caused by slipped disc
    or sciatica

20 × 30 cm (8 × 12 in) for back cloth; depending on **Size of cloth**
the condition it can be larger and about 20 × 60 cm (8
× 24 in) for neck and shoulder cloths.

Procedure The oil cloth over the neck and shoulders reaches down to the middle of the upper arm. The diagrams indicate how it can be firmly fastened to allow free movement.

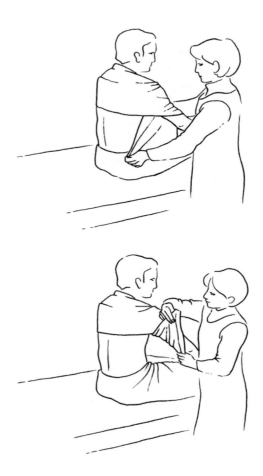

6

Ointment Cloths

Ointment cloths are cloths that have been spread with a plant cream, a metal ointment (containing metal) or a mixed ointment with plant and metal substances combined. This form of application is chosen if a substance is to be applied for several hours without additional warmth treatment. Ointment cloths are ideal for areas of the body that are sensitive to touch or for people who are very sensitive such as when experiencing pain or inflammation. An ointment cloth is used if the substance cannot be applied through rhythmic einreibung because of over-stimulation.

Different ointment bases are used for ointments made from plants and mineral substances because they each work in different ways and have a different effect on the body. When spreading an ointment on a cloth this difference needs to be considered. Mixed ointments can be spread like a metal ointment. Ointments are used in different strengths as indicated below.

Ointment cloths using metals and mixed substances

Metal ointments are manufactured to different strengths, and depending on the specific indication or condition of the recipient this is considered when prescribing. The most commonly used strengths are described.

According to the anthroposophical understanding of **Effects** nature and the human being, metals have a relationship with the planetary energies, human organs and their functions. The different metals are like gateways that allow the planetary cosmic forces to radiate their ordering formative energies into the appropriate organs.

The base of the metal ointments contains a substance that is not readily absorbed, for instance paraffin and Vaseline. This causes the metal ointment cloths to have a glistening, shiny layer from which the metal can radiate like a mirror on the part of the body being treated.

Metal foils Weleda in Switzerland make metal foils that are cotton cloth impregnated by different metals. These foils radiate the metal even more effectively. They can be lightly warmed and applied directly to the skin.

The length of application depends on the recipient, varying from half an hour to several hours.

Contra-indications Allergy to the metal substance or ointment base used

Weeping, infected skin lesions in the area of the cloth application

Material Prescribed ointment

Spatula or knife

Inner cloth of double layered material in the required size (2–3 cm, 1 in, larger than the area being treated)

Small plastic bag

Outer cloth that can be securely wrapped (may be firm fitting clothing or elastic bandage)

Hot-waterbottle

Preparation A thin layer of the prescribed metal ointment is spread on the double layer of cloth. Firm strokes are used to spread the thick metal ointment evenly over the cloth; it may take a number of strokes. It is important that the ointment is spread evenly flat and smooth, with a shiny mirror-like surface without any excess ointment. Leave the edges free of the ointment.

The ointment cloth can be used a number of times as long as the surface remains shiny. If the surface becomes matt or dull, then apply another thin layer of ointment until the cloth is shiny again. For the first few treatments reapply the ointment each time until the cloth is saturated. After this, the ointment only needs to be reapplied every 2 to 4 treatments.

Warm the ointment cloth in a plastic bag on a hot- **Procedure**
waterbottle prior to each treatment. Take the cloth out
of the bag and apply to the prescribed area of the body.
Secure it with the outer cloth or appropriate clothing.

1 to 8 hours as indicated. **Duration**
   In the case of a daily application, the treatment may
be given for two weeks.

Remove the cloth and replace in the plastic bag until **Finishing off**
next required. An ointment cloth can be used a number
of times depending on the type of ointment, the texture
of the skin and the body area being treated. Replace the
cloth if it develops an unpleasant aroma or seems to be
aged.

Quarter to half an hour. **Rest time**

Antimony and anise magnetised ointment on the stomach

Antimony or stibnite has the ability to stimulate life **Effect**
processes. Steiner suggested it is ideal to use externally
if the will is weakened.[1]

Metabolic weakness (gastro–intestinal mobility disorder **Indications**
caused by either the muscles or nerves that control peri-
staltic contractions) in patients, who often suffer from
sluggish digestion, with bloating and an unpleasant sense
of fullness after eating. Such people experience food
sitting too long in the stomach that leaves them with a
feeling of heaviness. Rudolf Steiner gave this indication
in patient profiles, suggesting that an antimony ointment cloth is applied in the evening remaining in place
overnight.[2]

This treatment is given after the main meal. The **Method**
strength of the ointments and drops being used as well
as the frequency of the treatment need to be decided in
consultation with the physician.

When the antimony and anise ointment cloth is applied to the stomach, give the patient 10 drops of chicory D3 (Weleda) in water, and again after half an hour to an hour.

Remove the ointment cloth after a further half hour to hour. Rest for quarter of an hour. The entire treatment takes 1 to 2 hours.

Caution This ointment is very black and discolours clothing and bed linen. For this reason use protective cloths.

Copper ointment (0.4%) on the kidney

Indication To stimulate the building up or anabolic forces of the kidney

Effect Copper is the metal of Venus. It is a soft metal of reddish, warm colour and has a full, warm sound. It warms and nourishes. A treatment in the morning can counter and reduce excessive destructive, catabolic daytime activity of people who are extremely nervy and rather weak. In the evening the treatment can help the soul to free itself of the body.

Steiner speaks of the relationship of copper to the formation of lymph and blood, processes that belong to the upper part of the lower body. Copper's radiating effect strengthens circulatory disturbances.[3]

Size of cloth About 20 × 30 cm (8 × 12 in)

Copper ointment (0.4%) on the upper abdomen

Indication Harmonising the parasympathetic nerve-sense system

Size of cloth About 15 × 25 cm (6 × 10 in)

Copper ointment (D3) on the feet and zinc ointment (D3) on the head

Multiple sclerosis.   **Indication**
Rudolf Steiner gave this indication for a man aged 46
who still had a certain level of vitality.[4]

To enliven the nerve-sense system and the astral consti-   **Effect**
tution, even when paralytic symptoms may be present.
    Sulfur is used to activate the warmth processes in the
body, while the bitterness of an acid is used to stimulate
consciousness. In multiple sclerosis there is a weakened
connection with the astral body, leading to cramping
and loss of mobility.

The following treatment is given early in the morning   **Method**
before rising. The strength of the ointments and drops
being used as well as the frequency of the treatment
need to be given in consultation with the physician.
    Prepare copper ointment cloths for the soles of
the feet and a zinc ointment cloth for the crown or
forehead. On applying the cloths to the feet and head
give the patient 5–10 drops of acidum sulfuricum 5%
(Weleda) in 30–50 ml (1–2 fl oz) water, and repeat
after half an hour to an hour. It is important to take it
through a straw to avoid damaging the teeth.
    Remove the ointment cloth after a further half hour
to hour. Rest for quarter of an hour. The entire treatment takes 1 to 2 hours.

Gold ointment (0.1%, D4 or gold mixed) over the heart

There are a number of mixed gold ointments used such as those including lavender, rose or melissa.

Effect Gold, the metal we use with heart treatments, belongs to the sun, the heart of the planetary system. It has a noble lustre, is immune to outside influences and acts to restore equilibrium and fill the human being with light.

Indications Relaxation and inner harmonisation
Treatment following a heart attack
People who experience an agitated heart or anxieties, worry, stressful thoughts or disturbed inner balance that is especially associated with night time.
This ointment cloth is often used when going to bed or when symptoms arise.

Size of cloth About 20 × 25 cm (8 × 10 in)

Lead ointment (0.4%) on the spleen

Lead, the metal most widely used when treating the spleen, belongs to Saturn, the planet marking the boundary between the solar system visible to the naked eye and the rest of the cosmos. This treatment can help patients who are too open and unprotected as well as those who are too closed up in themselves, helping to find a healthy boundary. It may be used for patients with neurodermatitis, food intolerances or allergies.

Indication To stimulate spleen activity

Caution As lead is slightly poisonous it is important that this application must not be applied for more than four weeks before a break.

Size of cloth 20 × 25 cm (8 × 10 in)

Lead ointment (0.4%) on the head

Too great a sense of openness, disturbed boundary to **Indications**
   the world and others, difficulty in being fully present
   (treat over the crown of the head)
Child with a very large head, hydrocephalus or rickets
   — children with rickets often have a soft flat crown
   (treat the back of the head)
The lead ointment cloth is not applied directly to the
head with the ointment to the skin. Rather the ointment on the cloth faces away from the head and another
cloth is applied over it and firmly secured.

As lead is slightly poisonous it is important that this **Caution**
application must not be applied for more than four
weeks before a break.

Dependent on size of head.   **Size of cloth**

Silver ointment (0.4%) on the bladder

Weak bladder, incontinence either from old age or pro– **Indications**
   lapsed bladder following child birth
Children, who bed-wet or lack bladder control during
   the day (in this case hypericum oil can be applied to
   the inside of the upper leg)
Chronic bladder infections (cystitis)

About 15 × 25 cm (6 × 10 in)   **Size of cloth**

Tin ointment (0.4%) on the liver

Tin ointment given in the evening stimulates the building–up functions of the liver, and may be used, for instance, to treat congestion or chronic hardening. Tin, which relates to the planet Jupiter, is a soft, ductile metal with a crystalline structure. Having a low melting point and high boiling point, it has an unusually large temperature range in the fluid state. It creates order and form when processes are too fluid or if they have hardened.

Indication Stimulate the building up or anabolic processes of the liver

Size of cloth About 20 × 30 cm (8 × 12 in)

Tin ointment (0.4%) on joints

Indication Joint effusion as with degenerative illnesses such as arthritis

Effect Tin has the ability to balance the fluids in the body, where there is an overabundance of fluid in the wrong place, or where there is a tendency for drying out. In these situations tin is able to bring form and regulates a healthy fluid balance.

Size of cloth Dependent on size of joint.

Plant ointment cloths

Plant substances are absorbed readily through the skin and because of this they are mixed with a base that is also easily taken in by the skin, such as lanolin, beeswax and oil.

Allergy to the plant substance or ointment base used   **Contra-indications**
Weeping, infected skin lesions in the area of the cloth
    application

Prescribed ointment   **Materials**
Spatula or knife
Inner cloth of double layered material, 2–3 cm (1 in)
    larger than the area being treated
Small plastic bag
Outer cloth that can be securely wrapped (may be firm
    fitting clothing or elastic bandage)
Hot-waterbottle

A layer of the prescribed plant ointment is spread on the **Preparation** double layer of cloth 1–2 mm ($^{1}/_{16}$ in) thick. Leave the outer edge of the cloth free of the ointment. Depending on the consistency of the ointment and the nature and absorbency of the skin, different amounts of ointment are required by different people. The ointment cloth should only have enough ointment for each treatment, so that when the cloth is removed from the skin little ointment remains.

The ointment cloth can be used a number of times, **Procedure** reapplying 1–2 mm ($^{1}/_{16}$ in) of ointment for each application. Place the ointment cloth in a plastic bag and warm on a hot-waterbottle prior to each treatment. Apply to the prescribed area of the body and secure with the outer cloth or appropriate clothing.

    An ointment cloth is applied for at least 2 hours and maybe left on overnight.

Caution Do not heat the cloth much above body temperature, as the ointment goes rancid if overheated.

Finishing off After removal of an ointment cloth any extra ointment left on the cloth may be removed before placing the cloth in an airtight plastic bag for the next application.

An ointment cloth can be used a number of times. In case of a daily application, it can be used for about two weeks depending on the type of ointment, the texture of the skin, and the part of the body being treated. When the cloth has an unpleasant aroma or seems to be aged, then throw it away.

Rest time Quarter to half an hour

Henbane ointment (Hyoscyamus 5%) on the upper abdomen

Henbane (or stinking nightshade) is a poisonous nightshade plant. It has a balancing, relaxing effect on the solar plexus that is connected to the parasympathetic nervous system.

Indication Cramping and disturbances in the parasympathetic nervous system
Inner agitation in fatigued patients
Restlessness and anxiety especially at night
This ointment cloth is often applied prior to going to bed

Size of cloth About 15 × 25 cm (6 × 10 in)

Mercurialis ointment (10%) for infections

Mercurialis is especially used when there are acute infections, to stimulate healing and relieve inflammation..

Inflammations in the area of abdomen, for example **Indications** colitis, diverticulitis, appendicitis, pancreatitis, cholecystitis

Inflammations and infections on the skin, for example furuncles, abscesses, nail bed infections

Superficially infected wounds, such as lower leg ulcers

Mastitis in breast-feeding women, when it is applied either as a follow-up treatment or at night alternately with hot mercurialis compresses (in this case the ointment cloth must be disposed of after each use)

If a mercurialis ointment cloth relieves pain then it can be reused over a number days. In this situation, it is removed after 12 hours, the application area is left open to the air for half an hour, then ointment is reapplied to the cloth before replaced it on the wound.

Oxalis ointment (10% or 30%) on the abdomen

Indications Fatigue and constitutional weakness

A weak digestive system

A disturbed digestive system caused by nervous anxiety, for example spastic cramping like abdominal difficulties or conditions.

This compress is often applied after meals. It is also used when a moist warm oxalis cloth is experienced as unpleasantly cool.

Size of cloth About 20 × 30 cm (8 × 12 in)

Oxalis ointment (10% or 30%) on the upper abdomen

Indications Following a significant shock or traumatic experience

This ointment cloth is usually applied before going to sleep. It can be left on for the entire night and even applied twice a day.

Size of cloth About 15 × 25 cm (6 × 10 in)

7

Teas

Tea compresses are given as wet, hot applications. One of the only exceptions is equisetum (horsetail) that is sometimes given as a warm compress.

Preparation of teas for external applications

Use fresh cold water. Cover the pot while the tea draws or simmers. It is best to use freshly prepared teas. This is especially important with teas using flower heads because they contain etheric oils that quickly deteriorate. This is obvious when comparing the colour and aroma of a freshly prepared tea to one prepared an hour ago or earlier, or stored in a thermos.

Teas made from hard stalks, bark or roots contain stable substances that are released more slowly than etheric oils. These teas can be prepared 2 to 3 hours before required and stored in a thermos. The tougher and harder substances require longer and more intensive preparation time.

Normally, 300 ml (10 fl oz) of tea is adequate for a compress. This amount of tea allows an inner cloth to soak and be well wrung out with little extra tea remaining.

Note A tea for an external application is made stronger than
for drinking. Use twice as much of the dried plant and
allow to simmer or draw for twice as long.

Part of plant	Type of tea	Preparation *1–2 tsp of plant to* *300 ml (10 fl oz) water*
Flower *(flos)*	Camomile *(Matricaria chamomilla)*	Pour boiling water over flowers, draw 2–4 min
Leaf *(folium)* and young stalk *(herba)*	Wormwood *(Artemisia absinthium)*	Pour boiling water over wormwood, draw 2–4 min
	Yarrow *(Achillea millefolium)*	Pour boiling water over yarrow, draw 3–5 min
Aromatic seeds	Caraway *(Carum carvi)* — whole seed	Bring cold water to a boil with seeds, simmer 2–3 min, draw 5 min
	— crushed seed	Pour boiling water over crushed seeds, draw 5–7 min
Hard tough plant parts	Equisetum or horsetail *(Equisetum arvense)*	Bring cold water to a boil with plant, simmer 15 min, draw 5 min
	Oak bark *(Quercus robur)*	Bring cold water to a boil with plant, simmer 20 min, draw 5 min

Camomile *(Matricaria chamomilla)*

In earlier times, camomile was considered a common meadow weed, while now it is less common. It grows best in dry, light-filled areas on the edge of paths and in waste land.

Camomile has a shallow root and quickly develops a thin stalk, growing up to 50 cm (20 in) in height, with many branches. The green leaves are linear, pinnate and feathery, comprised of fine leaf veins, with no flesh. In high summer, camomile has many flower buds, with a sunlike yellow head and white starlike petals. It almost looks as if each flower has a golden crown on its head, the folded back petals accentuating the crown's striving to reach up towards the sun. Camomile absorbs the sun's warmth, transforming it into dark-blue etheric oil called azulene, which is found in the flower heads. Azulene is one of the most significant substances obtained from camomile.

During the flowering time, the lower leaves yellow and become limp and fall off. Shortly after this, the whole plant becomes dry and withered.

The fine feathery branches and numerous flowers radiate outwards in their light, warmth-infused surroundings, opening freely towards the environment. Camomile has a sunny, open disposition that gives the impression of being light, airy and weightless. The flower smells sweet, tastes round, light and soft, infusing rapidly throughout the mouth, then disappearing as quickly.

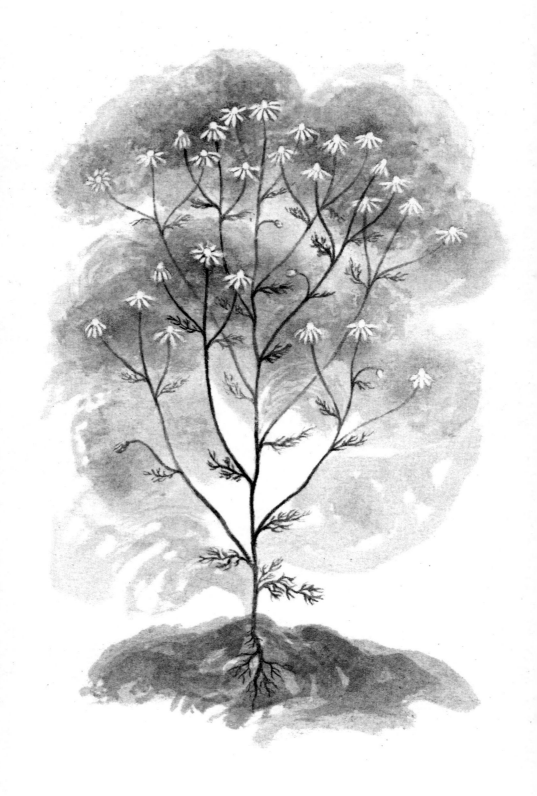

Through the camomile's internalised warmth, it has **Effect**
developed intense yet mild restrained sulfuric forces. This
quality enables it to be deeply warming and to release
cramps, digestive pain, bloating, nervousness, restlessness
and to calm troubled minds. Camomile also is used for
healing wounds and inflammations.

The Latin name for camomile, *Matricaria chamomilla,* is
apt as it originates from *mater,* meaning mother. This indicates camomile's calming, encompassing and comforting
properties, while being deeply ordering and healing.

Abdominal compress

Painful lower abdominal cramping   **Indications**
Stomach bug (gastroenteritis)
Anxiety and restlessness especially at night
Painful menstrual cramp
Unidentified abdominal pain, with a need for warmth
    such as hot-waterbottle
Chronic constipation
Nervous or hyperactive children, especially those with a
    tendency towards abdominal pain

Sudden abdominal pain with unclear cause   **Contra-indications**
Fever with unknown cause
First day of menstruation, as a hot application can cause
    heavier bleeding
Allergy to camomile
Skin infections or weeping wounds or cuts in the appli-
    cation area

Teaspoon dry camomile flowers   **Material**
300 ml (10 fl oz) fresh boiling water
Shallow bowl
Inner compress cloth
Wringing-towel such as a tea towel
Outer binder which reaches around the body, like a
    folded bath towel
Hot-waterbottle with a cover
Old face-cloth

Preparation Boil the water and pour 300 ml (10 fl oz) over the flowers, cover and leave to draw for 2 to 4 minutes. Fold the inner compress cloth and roll it up, place on the wringing-towel and roll the wringing-towel around it.

Put the hot-waterbottle in the middle of the outer binder (or bath towel) and roll the sides inwards towards the hot-waterbottle. Allow to warm for 5 to 10 minutes.

Procedure This compress can be applied soon after a meal or when pain occurs.

Place the outer binder behind the back of recipient, remove hot-waterbottle and have recipient lie back. Place inner cloth and wringing-cloth into bowl, pour (strained) hot tea over them and soak well. Then wring out firmly so as no tea is left dripping from cloths. Open the wringing-cloth and place the inner cloth quickly onto the abdomen, maintaining heat as much as possible. Place the face-cloth over the compress and wrap the binder firmly around the abdomen. Place the hot-waterbottle over binder in the required area. A knee roll can be used if required for comfort.

If the treatment is for a child, stay with them during the application time (15–20 minutes) and the 10-minute rest, perhaps reading them a story. Often these children will be able to rest and even fall asleep.

Duration Half to three-quarters of an hour.

Finishing off Remove cloths. Wash the inner cloth in warm water and wring out. Hang all cloths to dry.

Rest time Quarter to half an hour.

Caraway *(Carum carvi)*

Caraway seeds are rich in etheric and fatty oils, res-ins and coumarin (volatile active principle in plants). The seeds have a deep, penetrating warmth effect that releases cramping, shifts bloating and blocked air, and activates the digestive glands.

Stomach or body compress

This compress is made with caraway seed tea.

Bloating   **Indications**
Over-full stomach
Cramping in the digestive system
This compress is applied after meals or when symptoms are experienced.

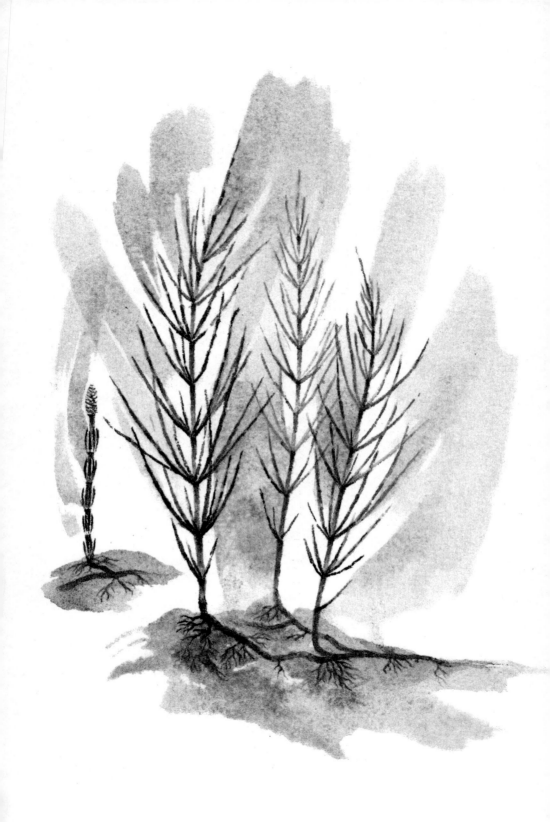

Equisetum *(Equisetum arvense)*

Equisetum or horsetail manifests very different plant forms at different stages. In early spring equisetum's flower forms; pale brown shoots form, 20 cm (8 in) long, with a cone-like bud at the end of a shoot. The tip of this spore cone has a six-sided shield around the spore dust. The spore dust can grow into new equisetum plants. As soon as the spores have dissipated, the brown shoot dies. The root stock sends up strong green fir-tree-like shoots up to 90 cm (3 ft) tall. The stem has a series of jointed segments that are easily separated. Groups of side shoots appear at the joints. Although the plant appears tough, hard and dry on the outside, it is succulent within the stem.

The root, often a metre long, is pencil thick and hollow. Because of the spreading habit of the root this plant is very invasive. Equisetum grows in fields, cultivated gardens, close to paths and dams, on wet, clay soils. The equisetum plant reveals a rhythm in the stem segments, has no leaves, little real root in relation to the stem size, and no real flower. The medicinal part of the plant is the shoots and stem. When dry they become a silvery green and are brittle, structured and formed.

The fresh plant reminds one in taste and smell of fresh, green grass. The dried plant has the aroma of hay and when chewed develops a bitter sweet taste that is hard to define.

In equisetum there are bitter substances, tannins and oxalic acid. The plant ash contains 97% silicic acid.

Effect Equisetum contains salt like, forming qualities that can be observed in its overly developed structure and high silica content. Because of these forming qualities equisetum is able to activate the nerve-sense system. Equisetum encourages structuring and is used to strengthen skin elasticity and connective tissue when there is excess fluid.

Equisetum also contains a sulfur component that enables the plant to form the reproductive shoot before the green plant stalks, and the plant contains sulfides and sulfates. The salt and the sulfur qualities interact in this plant. The six-sided shield on the spore cone is evidence of the typical forming tendency of the salt or silica, and the whorls of side-shoots show a sunny, sulfurous flower quality.

Rudolf Steiner spoke in a lecture about how in equisetum there are anabolic (building up) energies akin to those of the kidneys.[1] The kidney function can be activated by equisetum without changing the urine composition.

Depending on the temperature of the compress cloth or by adding a hot-waterbottle, we can use either the forming or the releasing qualities of the plant, as indicated below.

Kidney compress

Indications and temperature Chronic kidney infections to encourage kidney function (body temperature to encourage formative forces)
Bronchial asthma conditions (body temperature)
Kidney colic and kidney stones (as hot as possible, to encourage sulfuric, loosening forces)
High blood pressure with kidney involvement such as toxaemia in pregnancy (body temperature)

Time of application Usually done in the morning, as the kidney activity begins on waking and the compress can support this process.

Contra-indications Fever with an unclear origin
First day of menstruation as the hot application on the kidney region can stimulate heavy bleeding
Allergy to equisetum
Skin damage where there are weeping, infected skin lesions in the area of the compress application

1 tsp equisetum **Materials**
300 ml (10 fl oz) fresh water
Shallow bowl
Inner cloth (20 × 30 cm, 8 × 12 in) and wringing-cloth
Cotton or woollen binder (large enough to go round
    the body)
Safety pins
Two hot-waterbottles, 40°C (104°F)

For a full description see *Liver, abdominal and kidney com-* **Preparation**
presses on page 22. Boil up the equisetum from cold in
a pot with a lid, simmer for 15 minutes, then draw for
5 minutes. This long preparation time is important to
release the silicic acid.

Fold the inner cloth in half, roll from the outside
towards the middle, and put in a wringing-cloth. Roll
out the outer cloths behind the sitting patient. Place the
inner cloth in the wringing-cloth, put both in a bowl
and pour the prepared tea over them. Wring out well
and remove the inner cloth, which is laid on the kidney
area.

Depending on the desired effect this compress is
either body temperature or as hot as possible.

The patient lies down and the outer cloths are
quickly wrapped round and secured firmly. If needed,
place a warm hot-waterbottle on each side of the back.
The hot-waterbottles must not touch the spine, but lie
on either side of the kidneys. If necessary, use a small
roll or towel under the small of the back to ensure the
compress is firmly held to the kidneys.

Half an hour to an hour **Duration**

Remove cloths. Wash the inner cloth in warm water and **Finishing off**
wring out. Hang all cloths to dry.

Quarter to half an hour **Rest time**

Chest compress

Indications and temperature
Bronchitis with excess mucus (body temperature)
Dissipating lung infection, like pneumonia with pleurisy, pleuritis (body temperature)

Time of application
Usually done in the morning, as the kidney activity begins on waking and the compress can support this process.

Contra-indications
Fever with an unclear origin
First day of menstruation as the hot application on the kidney region can stimulate heavy bleeding
Allergy to equisetum
Skin damage where there are weeping, infected skin lesions in the area of the compress application

Materials
1 tsp equisetum
300 ml (10 fl oz) fresh water
Shallow bowl
Inner cloth (large enough to go round the body) and wringing-cloth
Cotton or woollen binder (large enough to go round the body)
Safety pins
Two hot-waterbottles, 40°C (104°F)

Preparation
For a full description see *Liver, abdominal and kidney compresses* on page 22. Boil up the equisetum from cold in a pot with a lid, simmer for 15 minutes, then draw for 5 minutes. This long preparation time is important to release the silicic acid.

Fold the inner cloth in half, roll from the outside towards the middle. Place the roll in the wringer cloth. The outer cloth is rolled from the sides to the middle and pre-warmed with a hot-waterbottle.

Method
Lay the outer cloth behind the sitting patient. Put the inner cloth within the wringing-cloth in the bowl, pour the tea over them, and wring out well. Take the

inner cloth out of the wringing-cloth and placed on the patient's back with the outer cloth on top. The temperature should be pleasantly warm for the patient.

If two people are applying the compress, they stand to the right and left of the patient. They roll the inner cloth out at the same time. Quickly secure the outer cloth.

If only one person is applying the compress, they roll one side fully out wrapping around and immediately covering with the outer cloth. They then continue with the other side. The outer cloth is firmly secured.

Lay a hot-waterbottle on each side of the patient.

Do not place a hot-waterbottle on the chest, as this **Caution** can lead to breathing tension as well as to a build-up of heat in the head. The patient must not under any circumstances become uncomfortably cold during the treatment.

Half an hour to an hour   **Duration**

Remove cloths. Wash the inner cloth in warm water and **Finishing off** wring out. Hang all cloths to dry.

Quarter to half an hour   **Rest time**

Wormwood *(Artemisia absinthium)*

Wormwood contains many bitter substances and this causes it to have a strong contracting effect. It activates gall bladder secretions and the digestive system.

Stomach compress

Indications Sluggish digestive system
Over–full stomach or nausea after eating
To activate the digestive processes of the bowel, gall bladder and pancreas
Gastroenteritis
Initial stages of migraine if nauseous or emesis
Relief of menstrual cramps
This compress is generally given soon after the main meal.

Method Pour freshly boiled water onto 1 tsp of wormwood leaves, draw for 2 to 4 minutes.

Stomach compress with wormwood and camomile tea

The indications for this compress are similar to the wormwood compress. The warming, releasing effect of camomile is added to the activating, toning effect of wormwood.

Yarrow *(Achillea millefolium)*

Yarrow grows in abundance in meadows and pastures, as well as on the edge of paths and railway embankments. It prefers sunny, dry and barren soil, and is very resistant to heat and cold as well as ongoing dry conditions, but does not like too much moisture. From the hardy root stock come numerous small light brown creeping shoots. The young plants have dark green, hard and somewhat rough, aromatic and feathery leaves, hence the name millefolium that means a thousand leaves. In the second year the hardy and tough pithy stem grows to a height of about 80 cm (3 ft), branching into a flower head, which has white or very soft, rose-coloured flowerets. Yarrow flowers from midsummer to autumn and often only the onset of winter ends flowering, when the dry stem can be seen to withstand the onslaught of frost and snow.

Yarrow gives the impression of being a very strong, down-to-earth, upright and solemn plant that is both held and balanced. It has a tangy, bitter taste, is aromatic and earthly dark. The tea tastes both bitter and aromatic and has a contracting effect, leaving a subtle aftertaste. The flower and leaves carry the etheric oil, azulene, which is also found in the camomile flower. There are also other bitter and tannin substances, as well as potassium salts.

In a lecture for farmers, Rudolf Steiner portrayed yarrow as a very special work of wonder which can greatly enthuse. Yarrow has an extraordinary healing effect, and he said it would be able to help the human organism from what is caused by a weakness of the astral body.[2]

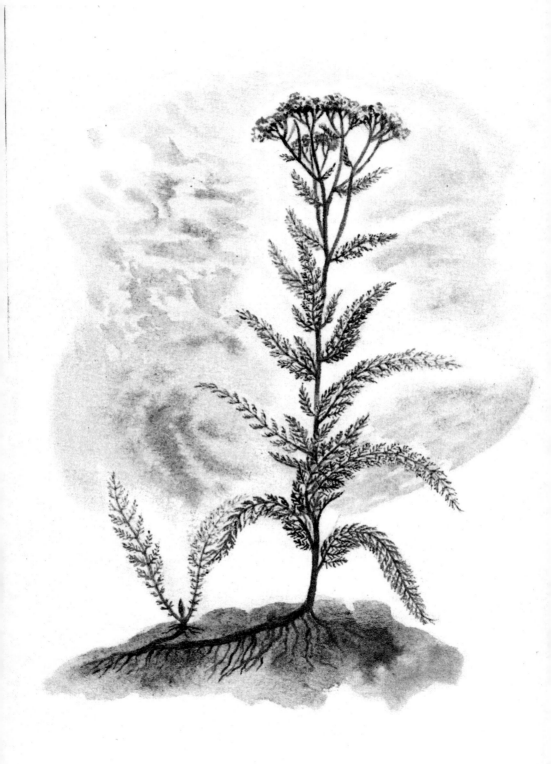

The sulfurous qualities allow a striving towards the cos- **Effect**
mos, openness, dissolving and loosening, while the salty,
structural forces hold the plant in a well balanced relationship. Therefore the effect is warming and loosening
cramp and tightness, moving excess air in the digestive
system, toning and drawing together, enlivening and
empowering. Yarrow increases the secretion of gall and
the working of the stomach and digestion as well as
animating the appetite.

Liver compress

Weakness of digestion system   **Indications**
To animate and increase liver activity after general
    exhaustion, the effects of antibiotic therapy or an
    operation
Depressive, 'out of sorts' conditions
This compress is ideally applied as soon as possible after
midday

Sudden unexplained stomach pains (an acute abdomen) **Contra-indications**
Fever of unknown cause
Cancer or metastases of the liver, unless prescribed
First days of menstruation, as a hot application to the
    stomach region can increase blood flow
Intolerance to yarrow
Skin wounds, weeping or inflammatory, in the liver
    region

In case of extreme tiredness and heaviness after treat- **Caution**
ment and rest (and if this happens after each treatment)
the application can be shortened to quarter of an hour,
or the compress applied without a hot-waterbottle, in
which case the compress is removed as soon as it feels
uncomfortably cool, usually 10 to 20 minutes, thus
causing a brief warming response.

Material 1 tsp yarrow flowers
300 ml (10 fl oz) fresh cold water
Shallow bowl and jug
Inner cloth and wringing-cloth
Generous outer cloth
Safety pins
Hot-waterbottle and cover

Procedure For a full description see *Liver, abdominal and kidney compresses* on page 22.

Boil water and pour onto yarrow in a jug or pot. Leave covered to draw for 3 to 5 minutes.

Fold inner cloth to 20 × 30 cm (8 × 12 in), roll towards middle and place in a wringing-cloth. Roll the outer cloth inwards and heat with a hot-waterbottle.

Unroll the outer cloth behind the patient who then lies down on them.

Pour the tea over the compress and wringing-cloth, and wring out. Take the compress cloth out and lay over the liver while it is as hot as possible. Quickly wrap the outer binders around the patient. Place the hot-water-bottle against the binders around the liver.

Duration Half to three-quarters of an hour.

Finishing off Remove the cloths. Rinse out the inner compress cloths and dry.

Duration Quarter to half an hour.

Notes

Chapter 1: Background
1 Steiner, *Man as Symphony of the Creative Word,* lecture of Nov 10, 1923.
2 Steiner, *Geisteswissenschaftliche Menschenkunde,* lecture of Oct 21, 1908.
3 Quoted in Grohmann, *The Plant,* Vol.1.
4 Steiner, *Spiritual Science and Medicine,* lecture of April 4, 1920)

Chapter 3: Cloths and Compresses
1 Steiner & Wegman, *Extending Practical Medicine.*

Chapter 6: Ointment Cloths
1 Steiner, *Introducing Anthroposophical Medicine,* lecture of April 8, 1920.
2 Degenaar, *Krankheitsfälle,* Case No 119.
3 Steiner, Introducing Anthroposophical Medicine, lecture of April 9, 1920.
4 Degenaar, *Krankheitsfälle,* Case No 125.

Chapter 7: Teas
1 Steiner, *Healing Process,* lecture of July 17, 1924.
2 Steiner, *Agricultural,* lecture of June 13, 1924.

Further Reading

Bentheim, T. van, *Home Nursing for Carers,* Floris Books, UK 2006.

Bühler, Walter, *Living with Your Body,* Rudolf Steiner Press, UK 1979.

Degenaar, A.G., *Krankheitsfälle besprochen mit Dr Rudolf Steiner* [Medical case studies discussed with Rudolf Steiner] Klinisch-Therapeutisches Institut, Stuttgart, Germany.

Fingado, Monika, *Rhythmic Einreibung: A Handbook from the Ita Wegman Clinic,* Floris Books, UK 2011.

Friedlander, K., *External Applications of Medicaments,* Mercury Press, USA 1996.

Grohmann, Gerbert, *The Plant. A Guide to Understanding its Nature,* (2 vols.) Rudolf Steiner Press, UK 1974.

Heine, Rolf, *Ingwerstudie – Praxisintegrierte Studie zur Darstellung der Frühwirkungen von Ingwer als äussere Anwendung* [Ginger Study: Integrated practice study on the early effects of ginger as an external application] Verband anthroposophisch orientierter Pflegeberufe, Filderstadt, Germany.

Holtzapfel, W., *The Human Organs,* Lanthorn Press, UK 1993.

Husemann, F., *Das Bild des Menschen als Grundlage der Heilkunst* [The image of the human being as a basis for medicine] Verlag Freies Geistesleben, Germany 1979.

Layer, Monica, *Handbook for Rhythmical Einreibungen According to Wegman/Hauschka,* Temple Lodge Publishing, UK 2006.

Pelikan, Wilhelm, *Healing plants,* Mercury Press, USA 1997.

—, *Heilpflanzenkunde,* Philosophisch-Anthroposophischer Verlag, Switzerland 1988.

Steiner, Rudolf, *Agriculture,* Rudolf Steiner Press, UK 1974.

—, *The Being of Man and his Future Evolution,* Rudolf Steiner Press, UK 1981.

—, *The Healing Process: Spirit, Nature and our Bodies,* Steinerbooks, USA 2010.

—, *Introducing Anthroposophical Medicine,* Steinerbooks, USA 2010.

—, *Man as Symphony of the Creative Word,* Rudolf Steiner Press, UK 1970.

—, *Nature's Open Secret: Introductions to Goethe's Scientific Writings,* Anthroposophic Press, USA 2000.

—, & Ita Wegman, *Extending Practical Medicine,* Rudolf Steiner Press, UK 1996.

Therkleson, Tessa, *Nursing the Human Being: An Anthroposophic Perspective,* Mercury Press, USA 2007.

Further information

New Zealand
Anthroposophical Nurses Association in New Zealand
PO Box 13001, Mahora, Hastings.
Tel +64-(0)6-844 5412   www.anthroposophy.org.nz/node/118

UK
Anthroposophic Nursing Association
Raphael Medical Centre, Hollanden Park, Hildenborough, Ton-
    bridge TN11 9LE
Tel +44-(0)1732 833924   www.a-n-a.co.uk

USA
Anthropsophical Nurses Association of America
1923 Geddes Ave, Ann Arbor, MI 48104-1797
Physicians Association for Anthroposophic Medicine (PAAM)
4801 Yellowwood Ave, Baltimore, MD 21209
www.paam.net   paam@anthroposophy.org

Index

RHYTHMIC EINREIBUNG

A Handbook from the Ita Wegman Clinic

MONIKA FINGADO

Rhythmic einreibung is a therapy of rhythmic body oiling. Its techniques were developed by Dr Margarethe Hauschka, based on suggestions by Dr Ita Wegman, the founder of the clinic in Switzerland which now bears her name.

Dr Wegman trained in Swedish massage. Rhythmic einreibung is a development of this which emphasises rhythmic elements and qualities which create lightness rather than pressure. The strokes work with the surface of the skin, rather than kneading the body as in traditional massage.

Featuring many practical exercises which help build up ability, this book is suitable for both beginners, and for those seeking to deepen their understanding of the techniques.

Monika Fingado is a trained therapist and worked for many years at the Ita Wegman Clinic in Arlesheim, Switzerland.

Floris Books